ALL WOMAN

In Remembrance

It matters not how long we live, but how.

'Festus', Philip James Bailey

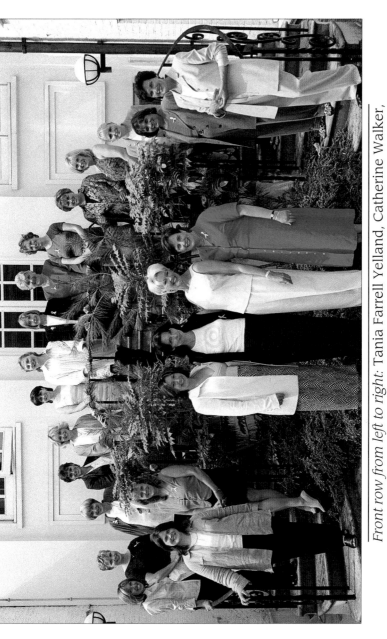

Front row from left to right: Tania Farrell Yelland, Catherine Walker, Diana Moran, Gillian La Haye

Back row from left to right: Delyth Morgan, Pattie Coldwell, Nina Barough, Fiona Jacobs, Judy Rich, Linda McDonald, Liza Goddard, Sheila Medici, Lolly Susi, Eileen Atkins, Shirley Harwood, Barbara Elliott, Pauline Silverman, Pat Leybourne, Elaine Tonks,

ALL WOMAN
Life After Breast Cancer

Compiled by
Tania Farrell Yelland

Photographs by
Arthur Edwards

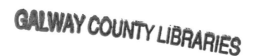

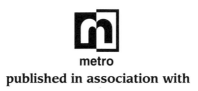

metro
published in association with

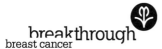

First published in paperback in Great Britain in 2000 by Metro Books (an imprint of Metro Publishing Limited), 19 Gerrard Street, London W1V 7LA
in association with Breakthrough Breast Cancer

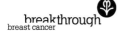

117,752

£12.99

Registered charity number 1062636

Permission to reproduce the following is gratefully acknowledged:

page 17: 'He wishes for the Cloths of Heaven', from *The Wind Among the Reeds* by W. B. Yeats © Michael Yeats; page 33: 'Snow' by Louis MacNeice, from *Collected Poems* (Faber & Faber), by kind permission of David Higham Associates; page 55: extract from 'As Sure as What Is Most Sure' by Gerard Manley Hopkins, by kind permission of Oxford University Press; page 87: extract from 'The Road Not Taken' by Robert Frost, from *The Poetry of Robert Frost*, edited by Edward Connery Lathem, published by Jonathan Cape, by kind permission of Jonathan Cape and the estate of Robert Frost; page 104: extract from *The Diary of Virginia Woolf*, edited by Anne Olivier Bell, by kind permission of Hogarth Press, on behalf of the Virginia Woolf estate; page 120: extract from 'Art and Public Money' by George Bernard Shaw, by kind permission of the Society of Authors, on behalf of the Bernard Shaw estate; page 130: extract from 'If' by Rudyard Kipling, by kind permission of A. P. Watt Limited, on behalf of the National Trust for Places of Historic Interest or Natural Beauty

British Library Cataloguing in Publication Data. A CIP record of this book is available on request from the British Library.

ISBN 1 84241 004 0

10 9 8 7 6 5 4 3 2 1

Typeset by MATS, Southend-on-Sea, Essex
Printed in Great Britain by Omnia Books Ltd, Glasgow

CONTENTS

PART 1: THE STORIES

PART 2: RESOURCE GUIDE

*The number in brackets indicates the age at which breast cancer was diagnosed.

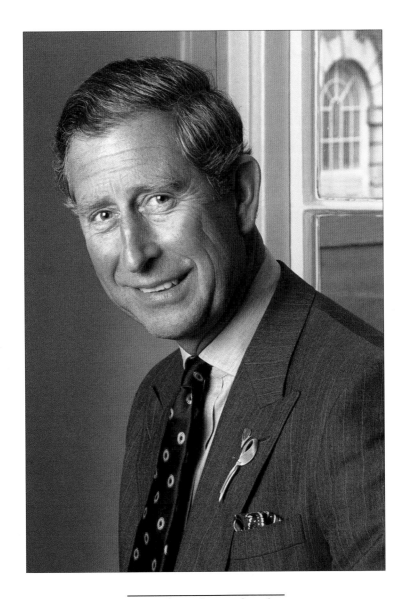

HRH The Prince of Wales

ST. JAMES'S PALACE

Like so many others, I have been profoundly affected by cancer through the experiences of my own family, friends and acquaintances, as well as through my own public work.

As patron of Breakthrough Breast Cancer and other cancer charities, such as Macmillan Cancer Relief, and through witnessing the work of the many hospices with which I am closely involved, I have seen the terrible toll breast cancer has taken.

While the statistics speak volumes, there is nothing like first hand experience to bring home the truly devastating effects of this disease. Every year, more than 30,000 women are diagnosed with breast cancer.

I believe the widespread effect of cancer on all of us can only highlight the importance of the many projects, and the urgent need for progress, on all fronts; research, diagnosis, treatment and care of those with cancer.

Because of this, I was delighted to become the patron of Breakthrough Breast Cancer in December 1998. In a relatively short time, a great deal has happened.

In December 1999 I was proud to open the first research centre dedicated totally to breast cancer - the Breakthrough Toby Robins Breast Cancer Research centre - in partnership with the Institute of Cancer Research.

The centre, near the Royal Marsden Hospital in London, is at the heart of one of the largest cancer complexes in Europe. World class scientists are carrying out pioneering research into breast cancer, bringing together different research specializations under one roof and examining closely both orthodox and complementary forms of treatment.

One of the keys to cracking breast cancer is, it appears, the greater understanding of what goes wrong with the genes in breast cancer. This approach will help to pinpoint new directions for treatment, new tools for diagnosis and even, perhaps, to help find ways of preventing the disease developing.

I have no doubt that a more holistic approach to these issues, making best use of the most advanced forms of science combined with complementary medicine and recognising that presently 'unknown' environmental or lifestyle factors may influence the development of cancer, is likely to be the key to success in this vital quest.

I am determined to help wage war on cancer in every way that I can and I have pledged that my Foundation for Integrated Medicine does all it can to help.

This book is an inspiration for each and every one of us. Every story on these pages is a tale of triumph, not only for the women who have shared their experiences, but for their families and friends who have lived through troubled times.

These stories show how each and every one of the contributors has continued to achieve in spite of breast cancer - or even because of it.

I am delighted that the book will not only be raising awareness of breast cancer, but also contributing to raising funds for Breakthrough and the Royal Marsden Hospital.

Research will help create a better future - but it is expensive. Now that the Breakthrough Centre is officially open, the challenge is to keep the ambitious research programme on track - a challenge with a price tag of £5 million a year.

Much has been achieved in recent years, as the tales and tears of these pages illustrate only too well. But there is still a great deal to be done.

I hope that this book will inspire you personally. For those of you who have direct experience of breast cancer or who have shared its effects with family, it will affect you deeply but, hopefully, instil a belief that there **is** life after breast cancer. For those of us who have fortunately not been affected by the disease, the recollections of these women will make you give thanks for your own lives and inspire you to live life to the full. For all of us, I hope it will add real meaning to the belief that research on all fronts offers the greatest hope of eradicating breast cancer.

Breakthrough needs your help to keep up the fight against breast cancer. It will take many years but it will take even longer if we don't start now.

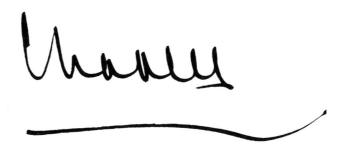

TANIA FARRELL YELLAND

The bravest battle that ever was fought;
Shall I tell you where and when?
On the maps of the world you will find it not;
It was fought by the mothers of men.
'THE BRAVEST BATTLE', JOAQUIN MILLER

Tania Farrell Yelland, 32, lives in Surrey with her husband David and son Max who is two years old. She wrote this book as a tribute to the many thousands of women who have heard, and will hear, the words 'I'm sorry but it's malignant. I'm afraid you have breast cancer.'

Wanting to dispel the myth that a diagnosis of breast cancer means instant death, she set about researching and talking to breast cancer survivors and specialist cancer doctors and surgeons, to uncover the real stories of women living with breast cancer. This book is a testament that 'we are healed of a suffering only by experiencing it to the full', as Marcel Proust put it.

Tania was diagnosed with breast cancer in 1998 at the Strang Cancer Prevention Center, New York, aged 30, and 18 weeks pregnant. She underwent a mastectomy and axillary clearance while pregnant, at the New York Cornell Hospital, followed by four months of chemotherapy at the Royal Marsden Hospital, London, after giving birth to her son, Max. She took tamoxifen for 18 months.

Tania's Story

When I was first diagnosed with breast cancer, a whirlwind of referrals and second opinions followed and a week later I was at the New York Cornell Hospital for a mastectomy.

It was all very harrowing at the time, as I was told I should terminate my pregnancy or I could risk losing the baby following the

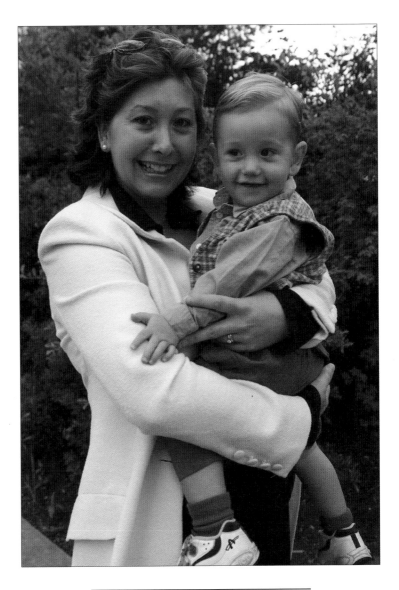

Tania Farrell Yelland with son Max

anaesthetic for the surgery. Fortunately, I did neither and I'm very happy to say that Max survived the six-hour surgery and was born four months later on 17 August 1998, five weeks premature, at Queen Charlotte's Hospital, London.

Max has been my motivation throughout this life-changing experience. When I was pregnant I knew I had to fight on for him. And after he was born, he kept me occupied so I had no time to feel any self-pity – especially when I lost my hair during the chemotherapy. In any case, Max, my husband (who has alopecia) and I looked like triplets with our shiny heads – which made a great photo opportunity!

During my time in New York, I had taken a liberal arts degree at the New School for Social Research. My graduation was in May, ten days after my surgery. But, not one for missing a celebration, especially one I'd worked so hard for, I proudly stood up with all my fellow students to receive my degree. It is a day I will never forget.

A few weeks later, at the end of May, my husband – a journalist – got a call from London, asking him to come back to edit the *Sun* newspaper. So on 1 June, another day I won't forget, five weeks after my surgery, David packed his bags to go to London.

It was daunting for me – left in New York alone, just out of surgery and 24 weeks pregnant – to pack up and sell the house. It was the most terrifying feeling to be on my own at night, not completely mobile after the mastectomy and not knowing how I would cope if I went into labour early. Fortunately, my parents, Val and Henry, as well as David's parents, Pat and Mike, came to stay over the next few weeks to keep me out of mischief. I am very thankful to them all for the time that they spent with me and for their help and support during my cancer treatment. At the end of July, I finally returned to London.

I was lucky because, although my cancer was very aggressive, it was detected very early and therefore there had been no spread to the lymph nodes. This meant that I could carry on with the pregnancy and wait to have chemotherapy after the baby was born. The fact that Max was born five weeks early was a godsend and it meant that I could go into chemotherapy a lot sooner – a week after he was born.

As Max was born by Caesarean, I was also able to have the very progressive ovarian cryopreservation at the same time as his birth, whereby part of my ovary was removed and frozen. This frozen section can be used at some point in the future, in a new form of IVF (*in vitro* fertilization) treatment, should the need arise. My frozen ovary section would be thawed, stimulated to produce eggs, which would then be fertilized and used in the same way as in regular IVF treatment. Cryopreservation can be performed as a precaution before cancer treatment is started as, in some cases, a woman's fertility is affected by the chemotherapy. By having this treatment, still in its experimental stages, younger women retain a degree of protection of their fertility. I was fortunate to consult with some forward-thinking physicians about this, before my treatment started.

I also sailed through the chemotherapy. I just got very tired but I think that had a lot to do with sleep deprivation caused by my new-born! The most obvious side-effect of the chemotherapy was losing my hair – which once you get over the initial trauma is actually quite a sensual experience. I will never forget the first time I showered with a completely hair-free head, or the times that David massaged my head to send me to sleep – sheer bliss! On the other hand, as I was bald over the winter months, I really know what it means when there is a chill factor. That's when I appreciated wearing a wig.

During my journey with breast cancer I have met so many wonderful people that I wanted to share some of their stories with you. There are so many women and men affected by cancer but we are always portrayed as 'victims' which is the last thing you could call any of us. Indeed, this book could have been called 'Women Who Do Too Much'. All are so active and successful and have accomplished so much. Each woman has shown tremendous spirit and determination in the face of adversity. Not only that – they have done so with grace and courage. I want other people to be aware of that and learn from it.

It is also very important that any cancers are detected early, which is why women of any age are advised to check their breasts regularly for suspicious lumps. As you will read in the following stories, most of these ladies detected their lumps themselves and sought expert opinions. If they hadn't been so proactive, their cancers wouldn't have been detected and treated so early. It is this early treatment which has basically saved their lives.

Cancer can strike at any age and this is highlighted by the life stories included in this book, where cancer has been diagnosed between the ages of 24 and 61 years. Of course, breast cancer is most prevalent in post-menopausal women but it is on the increase in all age groups.

This is why the work of Breakthrough is so important. Breakthrough funds research into prevention and cure of breast cancer. As so many women's lives are touched by cancer – and so will many more be in the coming years – it is imperative that action be taken to help Breakthrough and other organizations in their fight against this disease.

I am often asked how I feel about leaving the United States – where I was diagnosed and had my surgery and where statistically I have a better chance of long-term survival – to come back to London, where I had my chemotherapy and where treatment and survival rates are considered poorer. All I can say is that I have had tremendous care both here and in the US. I am very lucky and very grateful to have access to the finest doctors in the world.

However, I do realize that this is not the case for many women who cannot consult with a cancer specialist and who are, perhaps, denied the treatment they require, owing to lack of government funding. This book is for them; to raise an even greater awareness of women's fight against breast cancer so that action will be taken; to generate some money to help fund the vital research; to provide some support and encouragement to other women, so that they too sail through their treatments; and to provide an inspiration that they can survive this also.

Tania's tips for surviving treatment

- I made sure I never had chemotherapy on an empty stomach.
- I drank litres and litres of water each day.
- I took as many recommended vitamins and supplements as I could, especially Alkyrol, a shark's liver oil which boosts your immune system, Maitake D-Fraction, a mushroom essence, which stops you feeling sick and also stengthens the immune

system, N-Acetyl L-Cysteine which detoxifies the liver, and milk thistle which repairs any liver damage that can be caused by the chemotherapy.

- ❦ I drank loads of ginger ale (anti-sickness) and champagne (not together!).
- ❦ I slept when I needed to.
- ❦ I treated myself to a facial or massage when I wanted to.
- ❦ And generally I had a great time with my husband, baby and friends.

Tania's book recommendations

- ❦ This one!
- ❦ I also found *The Breast Cancer Companion* by Kathy LaTour invaluable.

Dedicated to my family and friends, especially with love to David and Max

Acknowledgements

So many wonderful people were involved in this book and they made it a joyous project to work on. I would like to thank a few people personally.

HRH The Prince of Wales, for his compassion and energy that bring awareness to many great causes.

Delyth Morgan and her team at Breakthrough, including Jackie Graveney, Peter Reynolds, Rachael Collins, Stuart Barber and Lindsey Hinds, for allowing me the opportunity to put this book together and providing me with tremendous support and encouragement. It was a privilege to work with such professional and committed individuals.

Professor Ian Smith for writing his introduction to Part 2 of this book and also for his reassuring care and attention. Margaret Moore for passing on my many messages and every one of you at the Royal Marsden who do amazing things every day.

Carole Pugh for introducing me to some of the most amazing women. You have made this book so powerful.

Lorna Carmichael for her expert research skills and her ability to calmly juggle several projects at the same time; Glenda Mogg for going the extra mile; as well as everyone at the *Sun* – they have all provided support in so many ways.

Daniel Taylor and Tim Ross from News International and Alex Armitage from Noel Gay for securing the best possible deal for raising funds for Breakthrough.

Also thanks to Michael Osborne, MD of the Strang Cancer Prevention Center, New York, and to KC, LH, MS, HR and KRM.

Alan Brooke, Susanne McDadd, Mary Remnant, Becke Parker and John Wright from Metro, for taking this project under their wings.

John and Mercedes Kay for encouraging Arthur Edwards to take on this project.

A very special thank-you to Arthur Edwards and his team, for the fabulous photography. This project took on a life of its own when Arthur came on board. He made every one of us feel relaxed and beautiful. Arthur, you captured the very essence of vitality within each one of us and for that I am truly grateful.

And to all of you wonderful women who took that leap of faith and contributed such uplifting stories. I am very proud of you all. You have shown such determination, courage and spirit. Your stories will give strength and light to other women retracing your steps, on their own journeys. Each one of you has accomplished so much, with so much grace and beauty. You are definitely 'All Woman'.

To my family and friends whose support and encouragement I will always remember.

And finally, to Max and David. To David, for being my guardian angel – 'You are the sunlight through my window' – and for opening so many doors to make this project happen; and to Max for being the life inside me that made me determined to survive.

Keep your face to the sunshine and you cannot see the shadow.
HELEN KELLER

Here's to life and all the joy that it brings.

ARTHUR EDWARDS

I would like to thank Geoff Webster and my son Paul Edwards for all their help and encouragement. I would also like to thank John Kay and his wonderful wife Mercedes who got me started on this project in the first place.

I was immensely proud and privileged when asked to take the photographs for this book about breast cancer. My wife Ann is a nurse and has first-hand knowledge of women suffering from the disease and has often been the first person a newly diagnosed patient has turned to. Through Ann, I have learned second-hand of how these women have fought so bravely against this cruel disease. I felt that by taking photographs of many of the women featured in this book I would help to promote a better understanding of breast cancer.

As the *Sun*'s royal photographer, I have photographed Prince Charles on his visits to Breakthrough and I have never ceased to be amazed by the way in which the sufferers show such great courage in the face of adversity and such a positive spirit.

All the women I photographed for this book were equally courageous and they offer proof that breast cancer is no longer a death sentence.

DELYTH MORGAN

CHIEF EXECUTIVE OF BREAKTHROUGH BREAST CANCER

I am delighted to have been asked to write this introduction in the company of so many inspirational women.

All have agreed to share the stories of their own experiences after being diagnosed with breast cancer.

I have read each and every one, delighting in their triumphs, empathizing with their most difficult times, and never failing to be touched by their courage in the face of anguish.

I know from my own experience the devastating effect that cancer can have. In the 1970s, when my father was diagnosed with lung cancer and my best friend's mother with breast cancer, the 'Big C' was never talked about openly, least of all to the children. This left us surrounded by fear and ignorance at a time when we were most vulnerable. For me, this book is symbolic of how times have changed for the better.

All of these women, from vastly different backgrounds, have a common bond in that their lives have been changed by breast cancer. All are living proof that diagnosis of breast cancer is not the end and that there is always hope for the future.

This approach unites these women not only with each other, but with the philosophy behind Breakthrough Breast Cancer. Only by having such a positive attitude did the charity become even a dream for our founder, Bill Freedman. Bill and his children founded Breakthrough Breast Cancer after his wife and their mother, the actress Toby Robins, had died of breast cancer in 1986. Bill was determined that something positive should come of her death. He wanted to find a cure for the disease or, better still, a means of prevention. He consulted experts around the world – but felt that existing research programmes would not have saved Toby's life. A new approach was needed. And so Breakthrough was born.

The charity was officially launched in 1991 with the founding aim of raising £15 million to build the UK's first dedicated breast cancer research centre. The very idea of raising this much money to

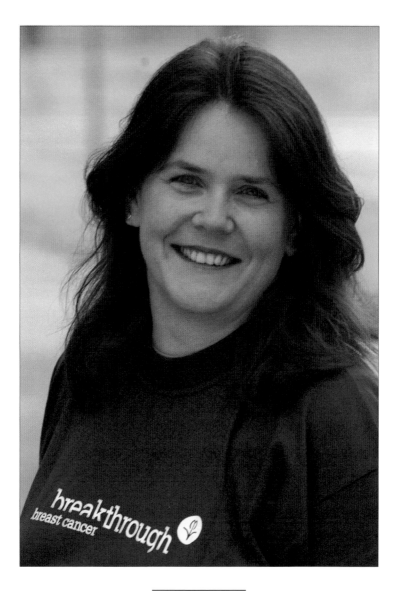

Delyth Morgan

establish such a centre was seen as incredibly ambitious. People simply didn't talk about breast cancer. That dream, shared by Bill and thousands of people throughout the country, became a reality in December 1999 when our Patron, HRH The Prince of Wales, opened the Breakthrough Toby Robins Centre in partnership with the Institute of Cancer Research. On that day, many of Breakthrough's long-standing supporters and newer friends stood side by side to celebrate an achievement that many may have doubted would ever be realized.

Why is the centre so vital? Breast cancer is a disease where the genes, which govern the behaviour of breast cells, go wrong. Only about 5 per cent of all breast cancers are hereditary and those are caused by mutations in the genes, known as BRCA1 and BRCA2.

Women with such genes have a very high risk of developing breast cancer. But what causes the genes to go wrong in the remaining 95 per cent of cases?

There are one million genes in every cell and 100 million million cells in the human body. Breast cancer begins in a single cell when the genes in that cell malfunction.

Technology has improved to such an extent that scientists can now work towards identifying and characterizing the specific genes involved in breast cancer. Huge advances have been made in breast cancer research over recent years but there is still much to be done.

Learning more about the genes involved in breast cancer and the biology of the breast is just the beginning. However, this knowledge will be essential in improving diagnosis and finding more effective and less harsh treatments for people with breast cancer.

Breakthrough is all about finding the cure for breast cancer. This is obviously the long-term goal, but research that we fund is also aimed at improving the quality of life of those affected by breast cancer and extending their lives as far as possible. The more we know, the more we can do to minimize the impact of this devastating disease.

The Breakthrough Centre presents an unparalleled research opportunity and a focal point for breast cancer research which should attract the best scientists in the field.

All of this has been made possible only by the 'can do'

philosophy that has always been at the very heart of Breakthrough Breast Cancer. Our symbol is the crocus which represents the dawn of a new life after a cold winter and captures the essence of Breakthrough.

Over the years, we have seen many thousands of pounds raised from the amazing fundraising efforts of groups, corporate supporters and individuals who have undertaken every conceivable type of activity.

The Breakthrough £1,000 challenge has captured the imagination of people everywhere who care about breast cancer. The many groups and individuals who have been successful in raising £1,000 are named on the Founding Wall at the Centre in recognition of their role in making this a reality.

In my four years at Breakthrough, I have been fortunate to meet many of our supporters who have achieved so much. Each and every one has proved beyond doubt that we can make a real difference.

I hope that the stories you are about to read will make you think about how out of adversity can come triumph.

Tania Yelland is to be congratulated for the achievement this book represents; no one is better placed to speak from a personal perspective. I know that this book will be instrumental in further raising awareness and ending the taboo of breast cancer.

Our vision is a future free from the fear of breast cancer. With the support of such women as those featured in this book, and with the magnificent fundraising achievements that never cease to make me proud, we can achieve that vision.

PART
1
THE STORIES

The eternal stars shine out as soon as it is dark enough.

THOMAS CARLYLE

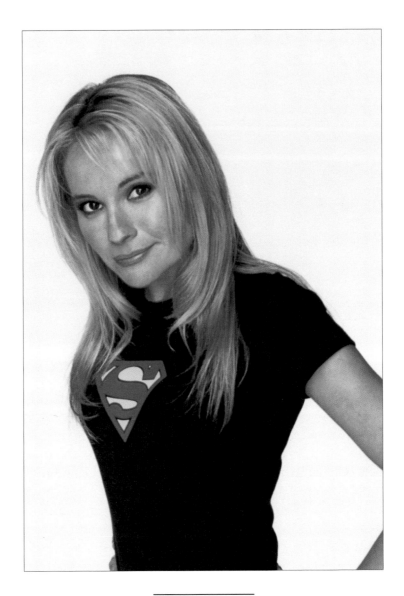

Belinda Emmett

BELINDA EMMETT

I guess I feel a little invincible, a little fearless. Once you've come face to face with your own mortality, day-to-day stuff seems a lot easier.

Belinda Emmett, 26, played Rebecca Nash in the TV soap *Home and Away*. She lives in Australia.

Belinda was diagnosed with breast cancer in Sydney, Australia, in 1998, aged 24. She had a tumour in her left breast with no lymph node involvement. She had a lumpectomy and axillary clearance with six weeks of radiotherapy.

Belinda's Story

I had basically been told I'd lost the lottery. I have no family history of breast cancer and the chances of it occurring in someone my age are about 30,000 to 1.

I had first felt a lump a few years before. It was only small and my sister had a hormonal lump so I figured it was something like that. Being 22 at the time, I didn't even think of cancer, I thought I was too young – I thought it affected older women. Later, a friend of a friend, who was only 24, was diagnosed with breast cancer and my friends and family pestered me so much that I decided to get it checked out for peace of mind and peace and quiet. I had a mammogram and assumed I'd be told there was nothing to worry about.

At this point I honestly didn't think about it much. I'd always been a fairly optimistic person and just naturally thought everything was going to be OK. I had a very hectic lifestyle and trying to fit in doctors' appointments was more of a nuisance than anything.

When nothing showed up on the mammogram, my doctor sent me for an ultrasound, which revealed a round, black mark. They thought it might just be a cyst, but I decided to go and see a specialist.

I had a core biopsy, which freaked me out a little because I suddenly started thinking, 'Maybe this is something.' When the doctor rang me and told me to come in and collect the results of the biopsy, I told him I couldn't because I was at work. He said, 'You really have to come in – now.'

I rang my best friend and flatmate, Kate, and she said she'd meet me there. The doctor told me, 'It's cancer,' and I just went numb. Kate was a godsend – asking all the right questions and listening to the answers. She was my ears because I really wasn't taking in anything at all. I guess I was in shock.

After a while, I was amazed at how incredibly positive and strong I felt. I was determined not to feel miserable or let it get me down. Looking back, I probably switched off emotionally and decided, 'This is a bit too tough, so let's not feel anything right now and just think about what has to be done.'

Focusing on life post-op, I opted for the lumpectomy with six weeks' radiotherapy, over the full mastectomy. Chemotherapy seemed more than likely and my lymph glands under my left arm would need to be removed to see if the cancer had spread. I had to wait four weeks for the operation and the worst part was having to drag that damn lump around with me. Despite my positive outlook and thoughts, I couldn't help but focus on that part of my body.

Although overwhelmed with support, I still felt a little isolated. I wrote down a list of things I could and couldn't handle and the two things I couldn't handle were the possibility of not being able to have children, and death. As chemo can affect your fertility I went to an IVF clinic and had some eggs removed and frozen. I didn't want to risk anything.

The night before my operation, I took my family and friends out for a dinner I dubbed 'the Last Supper'. As everyone was feeling as confident as I was that everything would be fine, my black humour was well received. That night was surprisingly fun and positive and the boob jokes were flying thick and fast.

I had to wait four days after my operation for the pathology results determining the severity of the tumour and whether it had spread. I was elated when my doctor popped his head around the door and said, 'I think you've won the lottery.' He told me it hadn't spread and that it wasn't as aggressive as they had initially thought.

It was the first time I had allowed myself to cry and, God, did I cry.

The chances of cancer recurring are slim, and physical imper-fections and regular check-ups are a small price to pay. I believe in fate and destiny and I think that's why I never felt the need to ask, 'Why me?' It made sense, it was a test of strength, a kick up the butt, a lesson to learn and teach. I was actually glad it was me and not a loved one – I don't think I would have coped so well.

You don't know how brave you are until you have to be, you don't know how much faith you have until it's all you have, you don't know how loved you are until you are overwhelmed with it, and you don't really know who you are until you're forced to look.

I don't want always to be known as 'the Breast Cancer Chick' for ever, but at the same time I don't mind being made an example of. Women need to know that breast cancer doesn't discriminate, anyone is susceptible. They also need to know that breast cancer is not necessarily a death sentence; early detection is vital, but there can be life after breast cancer and it can be wonderful.

I find myself seizing the day more often than not; I am well aware how beautiful and precious it really is.

Belinda's book recommendations

- *The Alchemist* by Paolo Coelho
- *A Guide for the Advanced Soul: A Book of Affirmations by Susan Hayward*

Dedicated to my family and friends for their constant love and support

Based on an interview by Rosalind Powell in *Hello!* magazine, 8 August 1998

MIRANDA VICENTE

It's OK to feel like shit.

Miranda Vicente, 32, documented her journey with breast cancer in the acclaimed Channel 4 documentary *Miranda's Chest*. She currently works as an air stewardess and lives in London with her two children, Daniela, 9, and Sergio, 7½.

Miranda was diagnosed with breast cancer in 1992, aged 24, while living in Spain with her (now ex-) husband and two young children. She had four months of chemotherapy before her first mastectomy and axillary clearance, followed by seven weeks of radiotherapy at the Clementine Churchill Hospital, Harrow, London. Eighteen months later she discovered a lump in her other breast and had her second mastectomy at the Costa Del Sol Hospital, Marbella, Spain.

Miranda's Story

When I was first diagnosed with breast cancer I had a four-month-old baby and a 20-month-old toddler. I was so busy and active with the children I didn't have time to think about what was happening to me. I think that this helped me in many ways. I was flying backwards and forwards between Spain and London for treatment so didn't have time to dwell on it. The more you dwell on it, the worse it is.

In the midst of it all I had a revelation one night. I knew I had to make a film about everything I was going through – it was as simple as that. I woke in the middle of the night and I remember saying to my husband, 'I've got to do this.' And that's how the documentary came about.

It took over two years to film, with the crew arriving every few months to stay for a week. It was hard going but everyone was very sensitive. I got to know them very well and they became part and parcel of everything I was going through with the reconstruction. To some extent it took my mind off things, especially when I was ready

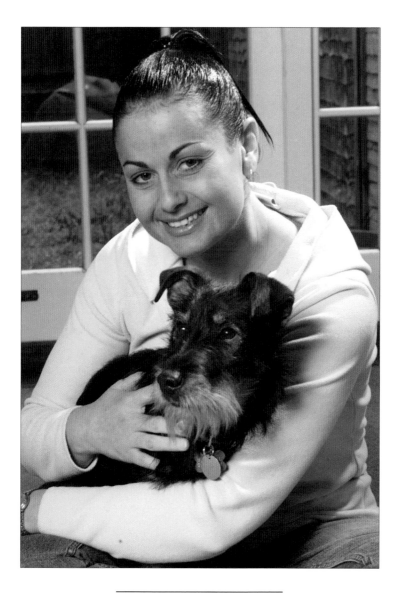

Miranda Vicente with Alfie

to go into the theatre for surgery. I would be talking to camera about what was happening to me. It sounded positive so I wasn't worried about what was coming next. It's my own personal diary of what was happening to me.

One thing I've always found about things you see in the media, such as TV stars talking about breast cancer or having chemotherapy, is how much pressure it puts on ordinary people. They say things like: 'I had chemo, I sailed through it, I was fine, I look great.' Well, when I went through chemo there were times when I felt absolutely grotty and I looked like shit. I looked in the mirror and said, 'I can't sink any lower – I've lost all my hair, I'm puffed out with steroids and I look like a wreck.' And it's OK. It's OK to feel like that. You don't have to be superwoman. Regular women with kids and money problems can't look like the stars. But you do what you have to do. Women do have an inner strength to cope and deal with these things – juggling lots of things all the time.

You have to cope with it in the way that you feel is best – you deal with it the way you want to deal with it. Don't be pushed around. Try to be positive. Try to see the end of the road. It often seems like you are never going to get there, but there is an end to the road. You might feel awful on the way – but you do get there and you do get through it.

When you go through an experience – any experience in life that is quite dramatic – you don't realize at the time how tense it is. I think after it's all over you realize that your life will never be the same again. It's certainly changed the person I am – it's changed my character. My tolerance level is zero; I no longer suffer fools gladly; I won't put up with rubbish. As you get older you also get more confident. Illness makes you think, 'Well, if I've gone through all that and I've survived it, there's no way I'm going to be pushed around by anyone or anything.' It changes your life gradually. It's a slow process over quite a few years.

My priority now is to be happy and content with my life. I'm always chasing some dream – I always think the grass is greener. I also have this niggling feeling that there's a clock ticking at the back of my mind – waiting to go off sometime. Life is for living, to savour each moment, to enjoy. I want my children to be healthy and happy.

As a newly single woman I thought I would have the most horrendous reaction from guys. When is the right time to tell a guy the whole story? Do you tell them the first night after a few drinks, 'Oh by the way, this cancer thing has happened to me and my boobs aren't real'? Or do you wait until later, until you're really into the relationship? Generally, however, the reaction has been great. It's not really a big deal to most men – which surprised me – they're really cool about it. It's probably me who worries about it more than them. It's actually nice to be able to start afresh with a new person.

I'm also not very good at trying to be something I'm not. I didn't think there was any point in pretending I had hair when I didn't. I lived in a small village in Spain so everyone knew what had happened. I didn't think it was necessary to walk around wearing my wig or wearing my prostheses, pretending I had breasts – when everyone knew I had lost them. It's a very personal thing. But it's OK to do what you think is right – there are no rules and regulations. And remember, you don't have to be superwoman.

Miranda's tips for surviving treatment

- Ask questions and be pushy.
- It's important to find the right doctor so go for second opinions.

Miranda's book recommendation

- *Love, Medicine and Miracles* by Bernie Siegel

Dedicated to my family – without their support I wouldn't have come as far as I have come. They've always been there for me.

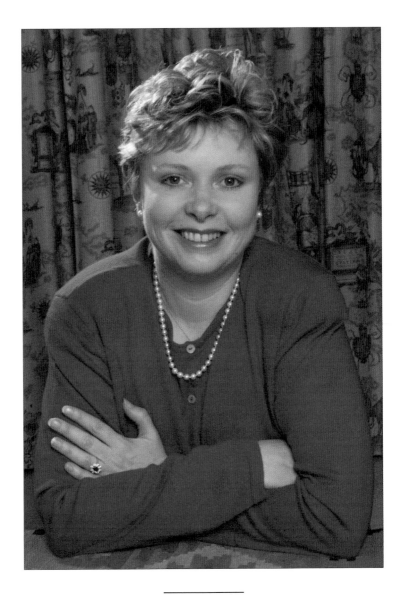

Fiona Jacobs

FIONA JACOBS

Something was missing from my work, my entire life in fact. Yet it wasn't wrong enough to force a change, until . . .

INGRID BERGMAN SPEAKING ABOUT HER HUSBAND, ROBERTO ROSSELLINI

Fiona Jacobs, 36, is a sales executive for a financial software company to whom she sold her own computer company following diagnosis. She lives in Waltham Abbey, Essex, with her husband Graham.

Fiona was diagnosed with breast cancer at St Margaret's Hospital, Epping, in 1993, aged 29. She had an invasive ductal carcinoma with two positive lymph nodes. Following a lumpectomy, she had six months of chemotherapy with four weeks of radiotherapy.

Fiona's Story

Looking back at the last seven years, I can quietly reflect that the fact that I developed breast cancer has changed almost every aspect of my life for the better – and that's a pretty profound statement to make. I know it is true to say that the most lonely and miserable time of my entire life was the initial impact of the diagnosis; the immediate treatment; the recovery period and, of course, the very early years worrying about recurrence; and subsequently watching friends made during treatment die. But the direct effect that breast cancer had was to change my life and me in a way I could never have dreamed.

The 'me' at 29 was married for four years, living a fast and busy lifestyle. My main focus in life was making a success of the computer business I had started with a colleague a year before.

Then it all changed.

When I learned I had breast cancer, the information was told to me gently but left no doubt in my mind that the condition was serious. I didn't ask, 'Will I die?' – that just seemed a stupid question once you are told you have cancer. I was more concerned with getting the 'thing' out so I could get back on track with my life. So initially I was very matter-of-fact. I absorbed the details provided to me on admittance for my forthcoming lumpectomy. The day came for the op and in true NHS style they didn't have a bed. I just wanted to scream at the lady on the end of the phone, 'Don't you realize I'm going to die if you don't get me a bed?'

Later that morning I was admitted. I felt strangely calm once I was there and just wanted my husband and my mother to go. There was a young girl of 16 having a lump removed and various other women having mastectomies and lumpectomies. It was like a club, everyone relieved to have someone to talk to who understood just how they felt. The only instant thing that struck me was how uninformed the other patients were. I had read up on types of tumour, survival rates, treatments, etc. Most of these women seemed to think that after the op, no further treatment was required and consequently seemed surprised that I was concerned about follow-up treatment.

I remember little of the six days I was in hospital, apart from specific incidents which had an impact later. One morning, an extremely ill old lady on my ward who had had an amputation of her lower leg hobbled over to my bed with a slice of toast, which she insisted I ate while she stood there. It made me feel like I was a pathetic wimp with no guts at all! It wasn't that she was lecturing me, in fact exactly the opposite – her care and concern made me realize that if she was willing to fight, there was no excuse for me!

When I was once again at home following surgery, the first thing I noticed was the rest of the world – a bit dramatic you may think. The day I got home, just for ten minutes we went for a walk in the forest. It looked so green, so alive and not at all how I remembered it. It even smelled different. People didn't seem to be the same either. The people close to me remained reassuringly unchanged but strangers seemed to be looking at me. I felt that suddenly people around me knew that I had had cancer. As a consequence, I hated being out or being left on my own. So my parents would arrive as my husband left for work in the morning. I wanted them there.

After my chemotherapy was completed, I took a holiday in Cyprus with my husband. The hotel we stayed in had a private beach.

One evening, there was a storm and the next day the sea was boiling up beautifully. Huge waves crashed down on the beach – it looked spectacular. So in I went for some wave-jumping. Then I lost my balance, slipped and came up to the surface a hundred yards from the beach. I started to swim back – I considered myself a fairly strong swimmer – but the waves just kept pounding down on my head. It slowly dawned on me that I was about to drown – the current was dragging me further and further out.

Not many people were about – no one, in fact. Then, suddenly, a couple appeared on the beach. By this time, I was gasping for breath and all I could think of was that I had fought to survive by having my operation, the chemotherapy and the radiotherapy and, after all that, I was going to drown! I was furious, so I shouted with all the effort I could muster and called for help. The man on the beach heard me and swam out. Fortunately, I didn't struggle and he was able to get me to the shore. The force of the water had pulled my swimming costume down and revealed my new scar. I know he saw it but he didn't say anything, he was just relieved to get us back.

I looked up the beach; my husband had been reading and had not seen what happened or heard my cries. I was in a dreadful state but the incident made me realize that God didn't want me just yet and had proved it to me in a way I had not expected. After the holiday I went back to work with a weight lifted from my shoulders. It was time to get on with my life and look forward to living.

The details of the failure of my first marriage are hardly relevant. I have now found a man who loves me in the way I need to be loved, who is always there when I go to the hospital for check-ups, always reassures me on down days, but is never unrealistic if there is a problem and constantly keeps ahead of what vitamins and minerals I should be taking to give me every chance.

He encouraged me to meet with my consultant and understand the complexities of the condition I had: why I wasn't taking tamoxifen (because my tumour is not oestrogen-receptive); and the possibility of our having children. I'm pleased to say that this was an extremely useful and informative meeting.

Once I was on the warpath of life, I decided to pick up a hobby from childhood – horse riding (much to my family's disapproval, mainly because the radiotherapy had weakened my arm and still causes me some discomfort which also affects my back). I took lessons and, three years later, Graham encouraged me to indulge my passion and buy my own horse. Chance (he nearly didn't make it when he was born, hence his name) is now six, and together we've grown as a team. We don't do anything very adventurous but it is something I do especially for me. We were complete opposites initially: he was fast, young, fearless and full of life, while I was cautious, old before my time and wondering just how much life was left in me! He gave me something else to think about. I knew he needed my help as much as I need his. He has calmed down and I am more confident, not just about riding but about everything.

I do often think how I would feel if the cancer returned. Of course, it is still a fear, but if I had all the people around me who contributed so much before and continue to do so, I have the comfort of knowing I could go through the challenge again. The whole episode completely reshaped my life, in my opinion for the better. I would hope that anyone experiencing either initial diagnosis or treatment might read this and think, 'I'm just like this woman and if she can do it, so can I!' After all, whatever life throws at us – illness, death, divorce, a house-move, whatever – how many of us give up?

So here I am seven years on from my operation. I remarried in April 2000 and I am a well and very happy and contented person!

Fiona's tips for surviving treatment

- ✿ Learn about what is happening to you and look after yourself.
- ✿ Self-help books can be informative.
- ✿ Visits to an acupuncturist are very relaxing.

Fiona's book recommendation

- ✿ *You Can Heal Your Life* by Louise Hay

Dedicated to everyone who helped me then and continues to help me even now

SHEILA MEDICI

Our deepest fear is not that we are inadequate. Our deepest fear is that we are powerful beyond measure. It is our light, not our darkness, that most frightens us. We ask ourselves, who am I to be brilliant, gorgeous, talented and fabulous? Actually, who are we not to be . . .? Your playing small doesn't serve the world. There's nothing enlightened about shrinking so that other people won't feel insecure around you. We were born to make manifest the life and light that is within us. It's not just in some of us; it's in everyone. And as we let our own light shine, we unconsciously give other people permission to do the same. As we are liberated from our own fear, our presence automatically liberates others.

<small>NELSON MANDELA</small>

Sheila Medici, 40, is a lecturer in English Literature, Communications and Philosophy at a college of further education. She lives in Epsom, Surrey, with her husband Noel and their two sons, Matt, 13, and Tim, 10.

Sheila was diagnosed with breast cancer in 1990, aged 30, at the Nuffield Hospital, Brentwood, Essex. Her original diagnosis was a non-invasive tumour for which she received a lumpectomy followed by a mastectomy. In 1992, she had a recurrence when it was discovered that all her lymph nodes were positive. She had axillary clearance on her left side and was given a 30 per cent chance of five-year survival. This was followed by six months of chemotherapy and twelve weeks of radiotherapy at Centre René Huguenin, St Cloud, Paris.

Sheila's Story

The Life of a Butterfly Who Flew in the Dark

The diagnosis story is simple, of course – unique – and it changed my life for ever. I went to the appointment feeling quite calm. I didn't even have my husband with me, but I did have my three-year-old son. I had left my baby at home with my mother who was visiting from Ireland. I vividly remember that Matt was sitting on my lap eating custard creams, covering me with crumbs and offering me bits of half-eaten soggy biscuit, in the way only toddlers know how. I haven't been able to buy or eat custard creams since. Anyway, there it was, the diagnosis: breast cancer. We took each day at a time and dealt with whatever was hurled at us. I have had recurrences and they too have been dealt with on a day-to-day basis, with a sense of humour and a stab in the heart. There is little point in pretending that 'everything is rosy now'. It hurts; each time it hurts. It scars; it faces you with a bitter-sweet taste of your own mortality; and the rest of the world carries on oblivious. I was given a 30 per cent chance of five-year survival – what a mess! But *they* were wrong, *they* didn't realize who *they* were dealing with – it would take more than a few cancer cells to beat Sheila.

During my cocktail of treatments, I found that emotionally and spiritually I was more attuned to my inner voices and intuition, becoming more introspective. For probably the first time in my life, my long-held beliefs were questioned, held up to a harsh light and examined. This was not in a particularly religious sense, although that was part of the process, but it was more of an acceptance of being part of an intricate and delicate web, over which I had little or no control. Recently I read a piece from *The Structure of Delight* by Nelson Zink. I opened the book randomly and found a short passage that matched exactly how I felt about life during and after my illness. The passage describes how moths instinctively are attracted to the light, whatever source it comes from. By identifying myself with something in nature – a moth – I found a waterfall of images from which I could draw strength and quench my thirst for peace and calm.

Very often at night, when the house was quiet and I wouldn't be 'found', I would stand and watch moths flitting around outside the window. The window framed the world outside and all it had to offer, if only I was brave enough to accept without questioning my part in the intricate web of the future. What intrigued me most about the moths was that sometimes one would alight without a sound and delicately pulse its wings. The others, crazier and manic with no sense of direction or purpose, would fly in circles, banging their fragile bodies against the tough, cold glass.

Sometimes, when a special moth alighted, delicate and shy, I would watch the light reflect from its crystalline eyes. The intensity of the light from its eyes was in sharp contrast to its dull colour. I would lean my head against the cool window and imagine that I could just make out the tiny movements of noiseless breathing. The special moth had consciously chosen to cease aimlessly flying in circles without direction. Instead, it had chosen to alight and, for a moment, just to *be*. This was not 'giving up', it was taking control of its own direction and focus of energy.

Lying in the dark, I would imagine that I could feel the flow of air from the calm, delicate moths with the shining eyes gliding through the darkness – the butterflies of the night. The image flows further with the words from Yeats's poem 'He Wishes for the Cloths of Heaven':

Had I the heavens' embroidered cloths,
Enwrought with golden and silver light,
The blue and the dim and dark cloths
Of night and light and the half-light,
I would spread the cloths under your feet:
But I, being poor, have only my dreams;
I have spread my dreams under your feet;
Tread softly because you tread on my dreams.
(The Wind Among the Reeds, 1899)

The butterfly of the night glides through the embroidered cloths of heaven – 'Tread softly because you tread on my dreams.' Still today, in my quiet moments of reflection, alone in the darkness of the unknown where I won't be found, I feel just like this, a butterfly of the night. I treasure my dreams.

There is something so very comforting in recognizing a symbol or metaphor for an experience, or for what one is becoming because of a traumatic change in life. It is especially helpful to identify a metaphor if the change is sudden and somehow out of one's control. Out of the ugliness of the chrysalis and the suspended animation, a new life, a changed being emerges. From the ugliness of the all-enveloping cocoon of cancer I emerged from the experience as a changed person in a positive and passionate way, who isn't afraid to dream or try the impossible. At epiphanic moments, another symbol takes over from the moth, that of a colourful butterfly of the day, rather than a dull-coloured moth of the night. The butterfly is slowly taking over the original metaphor, as the metaphor itself is changing and adapting to new dreams.

I have always refused to be classified as a victim of cancer, or a cancer patient, or a cancer sufferer – I am Sheila, who happened to have an illness called cancer. I am a person, not an illness. Inevitably, the butterfly of the day asked herself, 'Sheila, what do you really want?' The answer even surprised me. I have always wanted to teach.

Never one to waste a minute of precious time, I enrolled at North East Surrey College of Technology on an ACCESS to Higher Education course for mature students. Returning to study after nearly twenty years would certainly put the cancer in its place. I wanted to pursue a goal that would focus my lust for life; proving to myself that I had the ability to succeed against all the odds. As a mature student, I felt that life's experiences could only prove an asset in the learning environment. My cancer was just a nuisance, everyone has something in life to deal with; I had to get on with it. I completed a full-time BA(Hons) degree in English Literature and Philosophy. Not wishing to stop there, I returned to college to take a teaching certificate. You see, my attitude has always been that the cancer would never win – never.

I have, stubbornly, never allowed my periods of illness to affect my studies or academic standards. In many ways, the management of cancer has forced me to focus and prioritize anew each and every day. I have a heightened awareness of the value and gift of having a second chance to study and a second chance for life. Each day I look in the mirror and ask myself, 'What am I going to do with this gift of another precious day?' I have a sense of urgency about life. I live in time and not through time. I never waste time. I am often far too passionate and extremely volatile, quick to temper but quicker to forgiveness. I talk too much and listen too little, have an opinion on everything, with a keen sense of justice. My sense of the ridiculous keeps me sane in a world of madness.

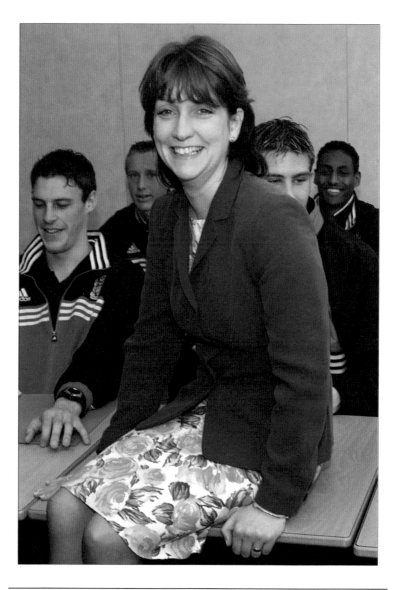

Sheila Medici with young players from Fulham Football Club

Ten years on from the original diagnosis, several battles won along the way, I can see that through the pursuit of my love of literature and philosophy, my outlook and horizons stretch far before me. I can now, just about, think in terms of one year ahead. Until recently, I still thought of life in terms of three-month chunks – the space between check-ups. I intend, next year, to apply for an MA, which I shall undertake as a part-time student. I am acutely aware not of what I do know but of how much I don't know.

I have returned to NESCOT where my adult learning started, this time as a teacher. I hope that my enthusiasm and love of my subjects will in some small way inspire the students to reach their own personal potential. Potential is just that, potent, strong, fulfilling and exciting. Too often I hear youngsters say that they can't possibly do that and then they learn how to do that thing they perceived as impossible. Empowering students to say, 'Maybe I could do that if I had a go,' and then watching them succeed is the greatest feeling for me as a teacher, and for them as blossoming individuals.

It is curious that I was asked to teach a group from the FA Academy of Excellence. They are the youth squad footballers from Fulham FC. It's curious because of my life-long boredom with and complete ignorance of football and because these lads aim for excellence in all things: their football skills; academic studies; and as ambassadors for their club. Although our experiences of life are poles apart, we have exactly the same stubbornness to be the ones to succeed against all the odds. There is no coincidence in this teaching-and-learning partnership.

I don't believe in coincidences. I have found that at the most difficult moments in life, usually out of the blue someone enters our lives to catch us when we are most likely to fall. Trusting my intuition to recognize and trust the Catcher is a lesson I have learned. I, too, am a Catcher and I am aware of my ability to notice who is about to fall. I try to alight and just to *be* so that I can catch them in time. We meet special people in the delicate and intricate web of life. Build up relationships and move forward because it is meant to be so. Because of my experience with cancer, I now know that my intuition is infallible and I live my life by listening to my heart and ignoring the logical advice of others. Pig-headed? Stubborn? Yes, I suppose so, but it works for me and I am at peace with myself and thus with others who function differently.

This is the Millennium year that I thought I might never see. The custard-cream son is a teenager, the baby is now ten. My family and friends saw, felt, heard and endured absences, hospital visits, moments of great joy and utter despair. Our sons have grown into compassionate, intelligent and philosophical lads who always think that they can do the impossible. They both have a most wicked sense of humour. My family has shared and faced up to the cloud that is cancer, with a deep wisdom and uncommon insight that few are privileged to have learned or experienced. Cancer may bring an end to an old way of life, but it can also be a perverse gift to a new perspective on life that so many, so thankfully, take for granted. So, next time you see a butterfly . . .

Sheila's tips for surviving treatment

- Don't rush. Have a second opinion. Ask questions.
- Be kind to yourself and the rest will follow – you cannot do or be everything to everyone.

Sheila's book recommendation

- *Jonathan Livingston Seagull, A Story* by Richard Bach

Dedicated to my Irish grandmothers – Sheila Clifford and Kitty Moloney – from whom I received wisdom, courage and a certain Irish something that helped me through with a sense of humour and a smile in my eyes through the tears

The quote by Nelson Mandela is from a speech quoted in the article 'Shine a Light' by Sue Knight in *Rapport,* the magazine of the Association of Neuro-linguistic Programming, Winter 1999, UK

117, 752

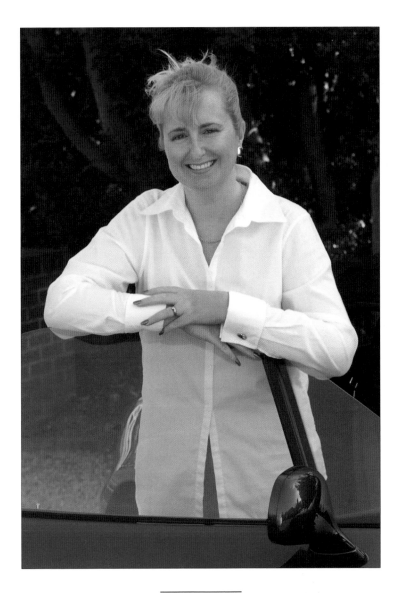

Elaine Tonks

ELAINE TONKS

We can't always choose the things that happen to us . . . but we can choose how we react to them.

Elaine Tonks, 38, has recently started her own company, called Blue Car Consultancy. She lives in Four Oaks, Birmingham, with her husband Paul and has two stepdaughters, Maxine, 21, and Jenny, 19.

Elaine was diagnosed with breast cancer in 1996, aged 33, at the Good Hope Hospital, Sutton Coldfield. She had a lumpectomy and axillary clearance followed by radiotherapy.

Elaine's Story

ET Finds a New World

On 12 May 1995, Paul and I were married in the grounds of the Almond Beach Club, Barbados, and I was so happy I cried. In February of the following year I started a new job and I vividly remember thinking that life doesn't get much better than this. I was 33 years old with a happy marriage, a wonderful husband, two beautiful and vibrant stepdaughters, and the career I'd always wanted. On Monday 4 March, I was diagnosed with breast cancer. I felt as though somebody had taken my entire world and turned it inside out.

To say that my diagnosis came as a shock is something of an understatement, particularly as I'd taken the day off work to have a tooth out! I had had a benign lump in my right breast for two years and for some reason I decided I would like to have it removed. As I hadn't been in my job long I didn't want to take any time off, but as I was going to have to lose a day anyway to have my tooth out (a particularly nasty extraction) I thought I might as well make full use of the time and go along to the breast clinic that morning to make a few enquiries. So that's what I did. This was on Friday 1 March.

The consultant sent me off for what I think was an ultrasound scan and the consultant radiologist said that she needed to extract a few cells with a needle. I thought nothing of it but what I didn't know was that she'd spotted another lump that was being masked by the benign one and she didn't like the look of it. The consultant (who at this stage knew nothing about the other lump) said they would be in touch to arrange the removal of the benign lump and, having sorted all this out, I headed off to the dentist.

Later that afternoon, the hospital rang and explained gently but firmly that they had some concerns and needed to see me urgently on Monday morning. They wouldn't go into details but advised me to bring somebody along for support, so at this point I began to realize that it wasn't going to be good news. Paul arrived home to find me crying (I was scared), bleeding (I had a great big hole in my mouth), dribbling (the anaesthetic was wearing off), and babbling incoherently about lumps. He guessed that there was something wrong.

On Monday we were told that there was a second lump, that it was malignant, and that I needed surgery as soon as possible. All sorts of thoughts filled my head. We'd been married less than a year and now we had this to deal with.

I'd only known two women who'd had breast cancer and they had both died.

How do you break news like this to other people? And on a purely practical level my private health care had ceased when I moved jobs and I hadn't sorted out new cover yet, so I was at the mercy of NHS waiting lists. I was on a probationary contract and would probably lose my hard-won job.

We immediately considered paying for private surgery (even if we had to remortgage the house) and then discovered that, despite all the horror stories we'd heard about the NHS, when the chips are down (or the lumps are up!) they really pull out all the stops.

My operation took place on Wednesday 13 March which, coincidentally, was Paul's birthday.

I don't know all the technical terms for my treatment so suffice it to say that the lump was removed along with eight or nine lymph nodes from under my right arm. We had to wait a few weeks to find out if the cancer had spread and I cannot remember being more relieved than when we were told that it hadn't. We cried more then than when they first told us I had cancer. This was followed by a course of radiotherapy, tamoxifen (for five years – only one to go) and months of exercises to regain full movement in my right arm.

So, four years down the line, how do I feel about all this and what difference has cancer made to my life? Obviously, given the choice I would rather that I'd never had the 'Big C' but, given that I have, I would have to say that it's been a positive experience. It has helped me to view myself, and all aspects of my life, in a funda-mentally different way. My priorities haven't changed but now I act in line with those priorities rather than just talking about them. My husband, family and friends now get the time they deserve instead of the time that's left over, and where I can influence the balance in other people's lives, I do what I can to help and support them.

Now you may be starting to think that this is a typical tale of career-woman-undergoes-life-changing-event-so-shifts-focus-and-career-goes-down-the-pan-but-she-doesn't-care-because-she-feels-fulfilled-anyway. But it's not like that. My career has gone from strength to strength since I was diagnosed. Not only did my employers not sack me but they supported me to the hilt and even promoted me six months later despite the fact that in my first seven months with them I'd had four months off sick.

Previously I had only ever worked in the UK but in the past three years my work has taken me to Chicago (nine times), Washington (twice), Cleveland (twice), New York (three times), Madrid and Dublin. I was a management development consultant operating as one of a team of three and now I lead a team of eighteen based here and in the USA. I've spoken at conferences both here and internationally and I've even been flown out to New York to do a one-hour after-dinner speech and flown straight back again.

During this time my organization has been going through a period of massive change and restructuring which means I've spent a lot of time operating in an environment characterized by both ambiguity and uncertainty.

I have no way of knowing what I'd be doing now if I hadn't had cancer but I am sure that I have been able to deal with many of these changes because of the way cancer has altered how I view myself and others.

For a start, my confidence levels have increased. Not because I think I'm better than other people but because I know that with their help I can achieve far more than I ever could on my own and, with my help, so can they. I would never have got through my treatment without the support of all those friends, neighbours and colleagues who rallied round. As I was somebody used to sorting things out for myself, that was quite a humbling experience.

I worry a lot less about things going wrong because I'm more aware that major changes in life, and work, can be waiting around the next corner and that you have to deal with things when they happen – and you'd be amazed at what disasters you can overcome when you have to. I've also changed my view on what constitutes a crisis and so am far less likely to panic. Consequently, I'm a lot more fun to live and work with, and I achieve a great deal more.

On a different level I've also learned to take time out to look for the joy and fun in life. On my first business trip to Chicago I drank a glass of champagne in the bar on the 95th floor of the John Hancock Center (one of the city's tallest buildings) and toasted being 'on top of the world'. Paul and I now throw a party every year for family and friends and each time we seem to have gathered more people around us.

The other major change has been that it's become increasingly important to me to feel that I'm doing my bit for other folks, and that's manifested itself in a number of ways. I raise funds for Breakthrough (£1,600 to date), support a mentoring scheme at work, and share my experiences with others who've recently been diagnosed and think that if you get breast cancer you die. I support a number of other charities including the NSPCC and Oxfam, and will also be doing voluntary work for the Breakthrough organization to help them with developing their people.

Now, before you begin to think that I've turned into St Elaine of Perpetual Positiveness and Good Deeds, rest assured that I also have some selfish moments. For example, my last car was a big saloon which came in very handy for ferrying people around, filling the boot with shopping, transporting bits of furniture from place to place, etc. My car now is a two-seater convertible – nowhere near as practical but much more fun and totally self-indulgent. I've joined a leisure club that I go to three times a week. I spend about 40 minutes exercising and then at least an hour lying on a lounger in a huge fluffy towelling robe reading magazines and drinking tea. Oh, and I have a manicure every fortnight without fail.

How would I sum up the last four years? I've learned a huge amount about myself and other people, and the great thing about learning is that (unlike lumps) nobody can take it away from you. I've also discovered that the world is full of incredible women who've beaten breast cancer but, somehow, we only hear the negative stories and I'm determined to change that.

On 12 May 2000, Paul and I renewed our vows at the Almond Beach Club and I cried even more because I have so much more to be happy about. I don't know what the future holds but so far things are looking very bright.

Onwards and upwards (or, as Buzz Lightyear would say, 'To infinity and beyond!').

Elaine's tips for surviving treatment

- ❀ Try to stay positive.
- ❀ Let others help you.
- ❀ Do your physio exercises.

Elaine's book recommendation

- ❀ *The Small Woman* by Alan Burgess

Dedicated with grateful thanks to Ian Paterson (Consultant Surgeon) and Bethan Lloyd Owen (Clinical Nurse Specialist – Breast Care) whose skill, support and capacity for caring have helped many women win their personal fight with breast cancer

SUSAN MILLER

We are still beautiful, we are still powerful, we are still sexy, we are still here.

My Left Breast, Susan Miller

Susan Miller, 56, is an award-winning playwright – winning her first OBIE in 1979 for *Nasty Rumors and Final Remarks* and her second for *My Left Breast* in 1995. She counts several screenplays and television scripts among her credits, including original feature screenplays *Blessing in Disguise* (Warner Brothers/Spring Creek Productions), *The History of Us* (Caravan) and *Becoming the Smiths* (Via Rosa/Fox 2000). Her television credits include *LA Law*, *Dynasty*, *Thirty-something*, *The Trials of Rosie O'Neill* and *Urban Anxiety*.

Susan was diagnosed with breast cancer in 1980, aged 35, at the Beth Israel Hospital, New York City. She had a tumour in her left breast and two positive lymph nodes. She had a modified radical mastectomy, performed by Dr Peter Pressman, followed by eleven months of chemotherapy. Susan lives in New York with her girlfriend Lida. Her son, Jeremy, 28, lives in Los Angeles.

Susan's Story

'Why don't you write about it?' my therapist said. 'You're a writer.' But *it* is many things. It is the time you've spent here and whether you are 35 or 50. It is who your friends are and how you see the world. It is whether you are someone who appreciates the irony or sees things in broad strokes. It is your style. It is your mother and father. The neighbourhood you grew up in. The passages you underline in the books you hold close. The surround. The interior. All the ways you were launched and where you went. It is what you hope to become. It is the list you make for the day. It is the history of you.

I said, 'I need a metaphor. I don't want to write about breast

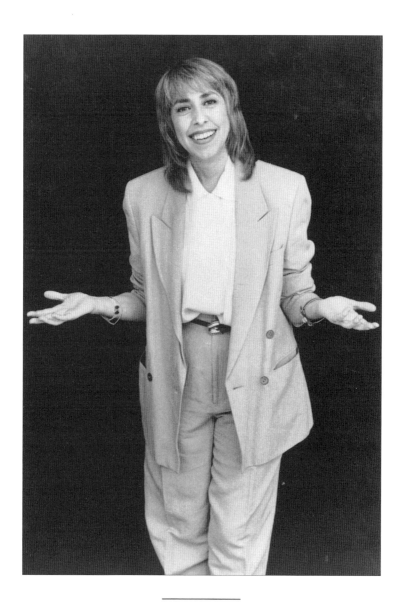

Susan Miller

cancer. I can't write about breast cancer. I can maybe write about a relationship I'm having. And one that is over. I can write about turning a certain age. I can write about being a mother. I can write about my son.'

And that released me.

It only took me fifteen years, but here's what I wrote.

Excerpt from *My Left Breast*

The year it happened my son was eight. He looked at my chest, the day I told him. We had these matching Pep Boys T-shirts. You know – Manny, Mo and Jack.

He looked at my chest and said, 'Which one was it? Manny or Jack?'

'Jack,' I tell him.

'What did they do with it?'

'I don't know.'

He starts to cry. 'Well, I'm going to get it back for you!'

Now he is twenty and I am still his mother. I'm still here. We're still arguing. He is twenty and I wear his oversize boxer shorts with a belt and he borrows my jackets and we wear white T-shirts and torn jeans and he says, 'Why don't you get a tattoo?'

'A tattoo?'

'Over your scar. It'd be cool.'

Here's what I wear sometimes under my clothes. (*Picks up breast prosthesis from desk and shows to audience*) Oh, don't worry. It's a spare.

When you go for a fitting, you can hear the women in the other booths. Some of them have lost their hair and shop for wigs. Some are very young and their mothers are thinking, Why didn't this happen to me, instead? (*Puts prosthesis in desk drawer*) And there's the feeling you had when you got your first bra and the saleswomen cupped you to fit. Cupped you and yanked at the straps. Fastened you into the rest of your life.

I miss it, but it's not a hand. I miss it, but it's not my mind. I miss it, but it's not the roof over my head. I miss it, but it's not a word I need. It's not a sentence I can't live without. I miss it, but it's not a conversation with my son. It's not my courage or my lack of faith.

My son did get it back for me. In a way. Not the year it happened. But the year after that and the year and the year and the year after that.

It was little league that saved me. It was Jeremy up to the plate. It was Gabriel Macht at second. It was Chris Chandler catching a pop fly. It was Jeremy stealing home. It was providing refreshments and washing his uniform. It was trying to get him to wear a jock strap. It was screaming, 'Batter! Batter! Batter!' It was Jeremy pitching the last out with the bases loaded. It was the moms. The moms and dads and the coolers. It was the hats we wore and the blankets. It was driving him home from practice. It was his bloody knees. It was the sun going down on us. Watching our sons and daughters play and be well.

This was the cure for cancer.

I miss it but I want to tell all the women in the changing booths that we are still beautiful, we are still powerful, we are still sexy, we are still here.

I unbutton my shirt to reveal my scar as the lights fade.

For five years I've travelled around the United States performing my one-person play, *My Left Breast*. I've been embraced by women and men and young people, who see in it their own stories. It wasn't breast cancer I wrote about, after all. It was a life. It is a life. And it goes on. We go on, each of us, to see what happens next and how we meet it. We go on to make what happens next a thing we value. We go on to carry with us those who can't.

Susan's tips for surviving treatment

- ❧ Don't go it alone. Be with someone. A friend. A partner. A person who can take you home and who will sit with you in the waiting room.
- ❧ If you have questions about anything at all – ask. Ask the doctor, ask the nurse. Write down your questions beforehand.
- ❧ Take something to hold. A talisman. A photo. Something to keep in your hands. For comfort and encouragement.
- ❧ Don't be afraid of the other people in the treatment area or waiting room. Sometimes it's hard to look at someone else's pain or illness or fear, but if you can take comfort in everyone's struggle, it will give you strength.
- ❧ Try not to think of all the treatments ahead, but rather deal with one at a time.
- ❧ When you get tired, rest. But don't get scared by confusing the fatigue that comes with certain treatments as illness. Don't think of your treatments as toxic. They are working for you.
- ❧ Let other people who care about you care for you – let them know what they can do. Reach out to them when you need support or company or chicken soup or a good laugh.

Things that helped me during treatment were singing Broadway musicals with a friend; watching old movies; eating whatever I wanted; getting fresh air; looking forward to something specific; doing my work; my family; and always, every day, Jeremy, my son.

Susan's book recommendations

- ❧ *The Stone Diaries* by Carol Shields
- ❧ *The Gold Cell* (Section IV), poems by Sharon Olds

Dedicated to Lida Orzeck who has also experienced breast cancer in her life

FRANCINE STOCK

The room was suddenly rich and the great bay-window was
Spawning snow and pink roses against it
Soundlessly collateral and incompatible:

World is suddener than we fancy it.
World is crazier and more of it than we think,
Incorrigibly plural. I peel and portion
A tangerine and spit the pips and feel
The drunkenness of things being various.

And the fire flames with a bubbling sound for world
Is more spiteful and gay than one supposes –
On the tongue on the eyes on the ears in the palms of one's hands –
There is more than glass between the snow and the huge roses.
'Snow', Louis MacNeice

Francine Stock, 42, is a writer and broadcaster. Her first novel, *A Foreign Country*, was published in 1999 and was subsequently shortlisted for Best First Novel by the Whitbread Awards and the Authors' Club Awards. She lives in London with her husband Robert and her daughters, Rebecca, 8, and Eleanor, 5.

Francine was diagnosed with breast cancer in 1995, aged 37. She had an invasive tumour with significant spread to her lymph nodes. After a mastectomy and four months of conventional chemotherapy at Guy's Hospital, London, she underwent high-dose chemotherapy with stem-cell replacement, including periods of isolation in hospital. This was followed by eight weeks of radiotherapy.

Francine's Story

The first curious thing about the diagnosis of a serious illness is that it is both utterly terrifying and absurdly familiar. It is medical soap

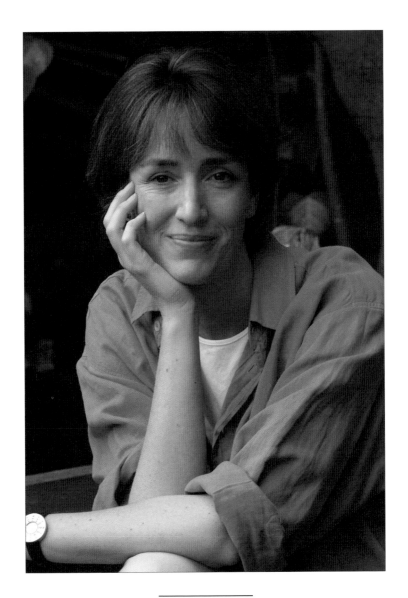

Francine Stock

opera come to life. Doctors and nurses can't meet your gaze; they fall back on their practised lines – 'There is no easy way to tell you this' – and you, the patient, hang there, numb and bewildered, your life suspended.

The second curious thing is that, from that moment on, nothing follows the medical drama format. Every dramatic cliché about the passive sufferer is wrong. Far from being simply The Patient, you are yourself, but more so. Illness is not a leveller, it accentuates the particular.

And life does change. There's no point in being Pollyanna-ish. It's not an experience you could ever welcome – but there genuinely are benefits from being forced to view your existence through the prism of emergency. All those 'maybe one day' thoughts crystallize into a will to do things today or tomorrow.

My life was hectic when I learned of the cancer: two young children (one of them a baby of five months); a job as a television presenter; and an outstanding contract to write a non-fiction book. In the space of a morning, all my obligations began to float, weightless, around me. The only thing I could concentrate on was the importance of staying alive long enough for my children to grow up.

Friends and colleagues were brilliant. Letters, cards and flowers began to arrive at the house. As my husband said, in the deadpan manner that he adopted for all our encounters with medicine over the following year, 'The great advantage of this over a fatal car accident, say, is that you actually get to find out now what other people think of you.'

Some friends or acquaintances simply phoned and came over – not embarrassed or constrained by the situation – with small kindnesses or jokes or practical help. People we had only just met invited us down to their house in the country to surround us with comfort and fresh air. I was so struck by the force of other people's good will – something that, in the hurried competitive atmosphere of the city, you often ignore.

There were awkwardnesses, of course. A couple of friends simply could not bear the idea, didn't know what to say and preferred to stay away. Others wrote of the tragedy of my situation. I didn't feel like a tragedy. I felt like me. Being a tragedy was somehow diminishing, even a little insulting. Even if I was going to die, I was going to live my life up until that moment in my own way – not like some TV mini-series mom or nineteenth-century heroine, quietly expiring, trying not to give too much bother.

After some painful early experience, I learned that research is good, but too much attention to media coverage of cancer is very bad for you indeed. There are always stories of people whose diagnosis has been more cheerful than your own and who follow exactly the same treatment – but who don't survive. Nobody ever bothers to write about the women who are quietly getting on with their lives decades later.

I also tried to avoid some of the survivors – the evangelists for particular therapies: 'You must have this'; 'The survival rates for that are so superior'; 'If you haven't had drug X you'll be in trouble'. And the Thought Police, too. 'Unless you recognize your pain,' said one woman who was convinced that breast cancer was a direct result of some repressed trauma in childhood or adolescence, 'unless you admit your pain in a group therapy session, then your cancer will kill you.'

Now, I believe that the causes of cancer are complex – and that emotional factors may well play a part – but I now reject any attempt to make me feel guilty. I was not responsible for my disease, even subconsciously. I will not beat myself up about it. I did seek counselling, but in my own way, and not as a result of being bullied.

But I did feel responsible for making every effort to make myself well.

If you'd asked me in advance if I would ever have undertaken such a drastic course of high-tech medical treatment, I would have been doubtful. I've always been a great believer in complementary medicine and the holistic approach. But this particular case called for total war. And while I continued to see a naturopath and aroma-therapist (the oncologist was always sympathetic to this), I also took the mainstream scientific route.

You have to devise your own personal survival plan – and leave yourself open to all options. No matter how weird something sounds, if it makes you feel good, do it. I became a great deal more tolerant – and consequently less scared of ridicule – during my treatment.

I was frightened of losing my hair at first – but when eventually it did go, I indulged in various wigs – short and sleek, long, red and rock-chick – I became more flamboyant, in fact. What I came to realize was that the inside bit, me, was pretty much constant and since there was all to play for with the outside, I might as well go for it. And when my hair came back, for the first time in my life I had curls, which was a novelty.

But the most fundamental shift was in my work. I had always wanted to write fiction; since I was a child, I'd scribbled away in notebooks. In my early twenties, I'd tried short stories – rather dark and obsessive – but had kept them, quite wisely, in the back of the drawer. But now, with so much uncertainty about my future, I knew that I wanted more than anything else to write a novel.

Sometimes, I did question the sense of spending hours locked in front of a word processor. Was I mad? Would anyone want to finish reading the manuscript, let alone publish it? I can't do justice to my sense of excitement and achievement when Chatto & Windus published the book, *A Foreign Country*, in 1999. It was subsequently shortlisted as Best First Novel for both the Whitbread and Authors' Club awards. I'm currently working on a second one.

I still work as a broadcaster, although writing takes up much of the time. After the solitude of the computer, I really enjoy the company in the BBC office. But if I stopped enjoying it, then it would no longer be worth the effort. Enjoyment and satisfaction are the real motivation now – career progression doesn't seem relevant.

Since my twenties, I've attended yoga classes in fits and starts. Three years ago, however, I began to work one-to-one with a wonderful teacher, Susanne Lahusen. With her help, I've worked on gaining balance and strength to redress the effect of the surgery. More than that, my body is stronger and better aligned than fifteen years ago. And I have one particular ambition, to do something that I have never had the nerve or the ability to do, even as a child, something that I always envied in others. By the time of my 45th birthday, I want to be able to perform – unaided, in the centre of the room – a handstand.

Francine's tips for surviving treatment

- My advice to anyone about to start a treatment programme is to ask as many questions, seek as many opinions and explore as many options as you can stand before you begin – so that you feel satisfied you are getting the best combination for you.
- All in all, my treatment took a year. That was bearable only because I took it each section at a time, with a generous system of indulgence and rewards built in – music, books, lunches, manicures, massages, films, holidays, whatever we could afford.

Francine's book recommendations

- *Original Blessing* by Matthew Fox
- 'The median isn't the message', an essay by Stephen Jay Gould

Dedicated to Rob, who was simply magnificent throughout

PAT LEYBOURNE

Life is not a dress rehearsal; always keep your options open and retreat with dignity!

Pat Leybourne, 40, is the Benefits Manager for Lichfield District Council. She lives in Rugeley, Staffordshire, with her dog Luke.

Pat was diagnosed with breast cancer in 1999, aged 38. She had a lumpectomy with axillary clearance at the Staffordshire District General Hospital and 15 sessions of radiotherapy at Stoke Hospital.

Pat's Story

I have always been an optimist and consider myself to be a very lucky person. I have lots of good friends and family, a good job, my own home and my dog Luke.

When I found the lump in my breast, I never thought it would be cancer. I knew I had to get it checked, and when my GP reassured me he thought it was nothing to worry about, I didn't. It was my friend Lauren who encouraged me to get a further check.

At the end of August 1999, I sat in hospital with Lauren, waiting for my results. I felt silly – this was not going to be cancer. I have a brilliant life. This couldn't possibly happen to me. So confident was I, that when the nurse asked if I wanted my friend to go with me to get my results, I said, 'No.' After all, I was going to be in and out in a few minutes.

The consultant was lovely – we chatted about my weekend. Then a voice popped into my head: 'She hasn't told you you're all right.'

'Come on then, what have I got?'

'I'm sorry, there are some cancerous cells.'

On Wednesday 1 September, I had the lump removed. When I

woke up, my brother John was there with Lauren. He'd driven 180 miles just to see me and all I could do was moan that I was hungry and thirsty. Tony, my boyfriend, had sent me a dozen red roses.

On Thursday, I couldn't wait to get showered and dressed. I congratulated myself on my organization of this. Shampoo and shower gel were placed in easy reach and my drain bottle was attached to the hand rail. Easy! One of the nurses found me a hairdrier. So I styled my hair, got dressed and put on some makeup. I had taken shorts and baggy T-shirts to wear. Unfortunately, the socks that I had to wear did make me look as though I was going to take part in a game of football – but it gave us all a laugh.

On Friday, the drainage tube was removed and I did a lap of honour around the ward. I stayed with Lauren for a week after leaving hospital but after that I felt that I wanted to be back in my own home with Luke. Concerns that he would be too boisterous for me were voiced but I was determined. Of course, he was as good as gold. He seemed to sense that he had to keep away from my right side and look after me. The day after I got him back we started to go out for walks, enjoying at least half an hour every day in the fresh air.

In July I had been to Turkey with five girlfriends. Despite living in Derby, my friends visited me in hospital. They took me out for lunches and shopping trips and thoroughly spoiled me when I returned home.

It was in Turkey that I met Tony. Tony is a big football fan. Personally, I can't see what all the fuss is about – it's only a game! At the end of September his team, Wimbledon, were playing Manchester United at Old Trafford. I'd promised in July that I would go to the match with my friend Lyn. So less than three weeks after my operation I was there, in among the crowds and enjoying every minute of it.

By October I was driving. I could get out and about to see more of my friends and do my own shopping. Alton Towers put on a huge firework display and Tony arranged for us to spend the day there with friends. There I was, less than eight weeks after the op, going on all the rides at Alton Towers just the same as I would have done before.

In mid-November my radiotherapy began. Someone somewhere had said that you could work through radiotherapy. I was going to do that too – I was desperate to go back to work. My treatment was on Mondays, Wednesdays and Fridays so I went back to work on Tuesdays and Thursdays. I drove the 50-mile round trip to and from the hospital every time myself. Sometimes Lauren gave me her shopping list and I would get her shopping for her! So within three months I was back at work, albeit part time.

The works Christmas party had been booked in April. I wasn't going to miss it and I had a new 'little black number' to go in. I was there until 2 a.m. – the bitter end. New Year – the Millennium – was also organized. That night I was in the pub until 3.30 p.m. and rumour has it that I was dancing on the table after midnight!

In January I began to build up my hours at work. By the end of January I was working three days. I also enrolled at the gym to start some gentle exercise, and I've redecorated my living room – with a little bit of help!

In February I was working and feeling stronger and less tired. My greatest achievement this month was wearing a bra all day. At this rate of recovery I would be in my Wonderbra in March!

On 17 March, my doctor signed me fit for work – after some arm-twisting and a promise I would rest. And I've started to take regular trips to see Tony in London where I always take full advantage of the shops!

I went to see the consultant who did my operation. He is very proud of his work and I feel that he looks at me as if I'm a portrait he's just painted.

I still believe I'm the luckiest person in the world. I caught the cancer early and now it's gone. It's been an inconvenience but I'm getting my life back and that's all I want.

Pat's tips for surviving the treatment

- Go with the flow but keep yourself organized.
- If you're tired, rest. If you're not – do those jobs! I used to prepare meals for the next day, so that if I felt especially tired after my treatment, all I did was turn the oven on.

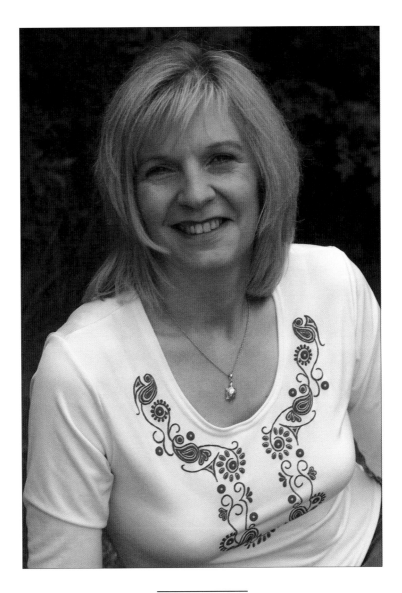

Pat Leybourne

Pat's book recommendation

The 'Harry Potter' series by J. K. Rowling

Dedicated to my friends and family. Friends at work, especially Sally who suffered my 'off' days; Jean, Angie and the Turkey girls for getting me out; John and Janet for the gorgeous gifts; Mum and Dad and Martyn. For Tony, whose caring support, kindness and sense of humour have been invaluable. And for Lauren, who has been through the whole experience with me. For all the time she has made for me – the appointments, laughs, cries and shopping – I couldn't have been positive without her. I hope that everyone has at least one friend like her.

GILLIAN LA HAYE

Value each day for what it brings; find the good in every situation; give as much love as you can to everyone you meet; get to know your God.

Gillian La Haye, 51, is a Bowen technique therapist – a non-invasive form of healing bodywork. She lives in New Malden, Surrey, with her husband Tim and son Nicholas, 11.

Gillian was diagnosed with breast cancer in 1988, aged 39 and four weeks pregnant with Nicholas, her first child. She had a lumpectomy and axillary clearance at the Clementine Churchill Hospital, Harrow, London, followed by 15 sessions of radiotherapy at the Mount Vernon Hospital, London.

Gillian's Story

This is a book to celebrate life. What I would say about this is not perhaps what everyone would want to hear.

Human life is the greatest gift we have – it is given to us freely. We long for it, we guard it jealously and we hang on to it frantically. We fear its loss. The gift of human life is for ever. It opens up the opportunity of real and total fulfilment and happiness in union with our creator, God. The God who gives us the most precious gift we have longs to share that eternal fulfilment with us and our earthly life is the journey we make towards that – 'talents' in hand.

What we make of those talents – the few treasures and tools we have been given to help us on that journey – is up to us. We may bury them and lie low; we may take them out every now and then, blow the dust off them, polish them greedily but put them away again when we realize that they may cause us to have to think, to work, to give . . . ; we may get up and run with them, work hard, use initiative, give of our best, but lose heart when the going gets tough and give up; we may, however, keep going through thick and thin, no matter what the cost, because we have understood that the more we give, the greater the return, the more we love, never mind the hurt, the more worthwhile life is . . .

Believe it or not, our cancer is one of our 'talents'. We have been entrusted with this difficulty not as some curse or some deadly enemy but as something with which to learn to love more, to give more than we ever imagined possible.

Isn't it true that through cancer you have met hosts of people you wouldn't otherwise have met? Why might that have been? Mere chance, coming out of necessity? Or perhaps so that your life's journey might affect them, might bring to them some joy, some wisdom, some knowledge, some depth, some friendship, some love they would not otherwise have had?

And you? Have you not gained from them so many pearls, so many joys, so much friendship? Have you not learned so much from the simplicity of their warmth towards you, from the generosity of their time, their wisdom, their love?

Isn't it true, also, that through cancer you have encountered challenges, experiences which would otherwise have passed you by?

Isn't it true that these experiences – difficult, tough, traumatic, hurtful, appalling though they may sometimes have been – have brought you a wealth of knowledge, of understanding, have knocked off your rough edges, brought you wisdom and hope and deepened your longing to help others?

If all this is true of your experience then you've been making the most of your 'talent', the very special 'talent' you most unexpectedly found in your 'toolbox'.

Many, many people have this talent. Most people have some similar talent, one that we would not choose, one which we do not understand, one which seems unfair. But if only we can shed the 'poor me' and see through the shock-horror, what a wealth of opportunity we shall find: opportunities to give ourselves; to be strong; to be wise; to be filled with hope and joy; to learn to be a friend, a real friend; to learn to love others for what they are, not for what we want them to be; opportunities to prioritize our lives; to see through the peripherals and trappings of wealth to the real issues of faith, hope and love – real love; opportunities to search within ourselves to find the real meaning of our lives; opportunities to seek outside ourselves for the real meaning of life and to get to know our God.

So yes, let's celebrate all that life is, all that life brings. Let us never fear what life may bring ever again because out there, there is a far greater meaning to it all. This is something which cancer cannot kill, and by using well this 'talent' which our cancer has been and for some of us still is, we shall enrich not only our own lives into all eternity but also those of countless others.

We shall never know in this life how many lives ours has touched but let us pray that whoever is touched by ours may be enriched and may feel the more love for having known us.

Cancer has given me an awareness of my mortality – I'm no longer afraid of death. I want to get the most out of every minute of life.

See this as the next adventure, the next challenge. Accept all the love and give all you can. Try to see this as a privilege – you are so special that you have been given this much, you are worth so much, you have been entrusted to take this. It's tough, it's a challenge, but you can do it. Whatever the outcome, you will have achieved so much.

Gillian's tips for surviving treatment

- Know as much as you can, find out everything you can about your case and what your options are.
- Seek second and third opinions. Take control.
- Share this information with only one or two people close to you. To discuss it with all the family causes confusion and too many 'helpful' opinions.

Gillian's book recommendation

- *The Way* by Blessed Josemaria Escriva

Dedicated to my son Nicholas, whose presence within me was the life force which spurred me on, and my husband Tim, whose love and total support were my strength

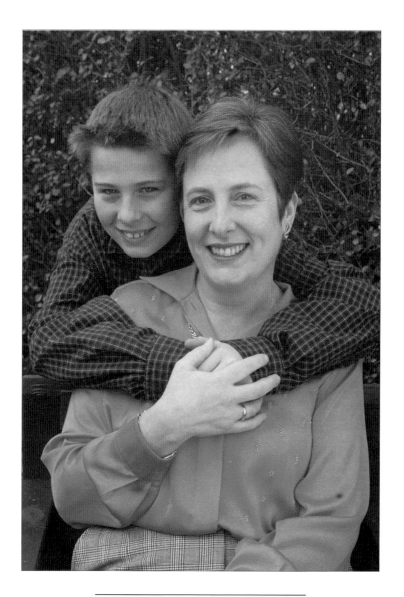

Gillian La Haye with son Nicholas

NINA BAROUGH

There is life at the end of the tunnel – exciting, wonderful life which you cannot see in the beginning.

Nina Barough, 45, is a fundraiser and event organizer. She is Managing Director of Walk the Walk, an organization dedicated to raising awareness of good health and well-being in all women and men. She lives in London.

Nina was diagnosed with breast cancer in Arizona in 1997, aged 41. She had a lumpectomy followed by a mastectomy and radiotherapy at the City Hospital, Nottingham. She also had zoladex injections and took tamoxifen for two years.

Nina's Story

4 January 1997
Flew out to Arizona desert to work on a Wrangler shoot

5 January 1997
Found a lump in my breast – panic – went to see a doctor

6 January 1997
In between working had mammogram

7 January 1997
Had an ultrasound – told to cancel everything – life stops!

Once upon a time three years ago, I was a photographers' stylist, a very busy, hectic stylist, rushing from one job to another. I was always very active in a busy, rushing kind of way, living a cocktail of hotels, studios, travelling and sheer adrenalin. My saving grace (or so I thought) was that I have always had an avid fascination with inner health and well-being so, although I did not have much time for myself, I ate well and I tried to keep myself fit. I have always had the belief that if you could find the magical and elusive balance within the mind, body and spirit then everything would be fine.

I arrived home from Arizona on a Monday morning clutching my X–rays and test results – by Saturday I was in hospital having a lumpectomy. One of the most frightening parts of being told that I had breast cancer was the speed with which everything happened. In just over a week I had gone from being this independent working woman to being a frightened and shocked person I could barely recognize.

My mum came to stay to look after me. Neither of us could understand why it was happening – this was something that happened to other people, not me. It felt as though my life had stopped, and in many ways, as I waited for my results, it had. But worse still, I didn't know how I could rescue myself.

'I am sure everything will be fine,' everybody kept telling me. I really wanted to believe that – to believe that any day now the phone would ring and the nurse would apologize for the mistake, but there had been a mix-up and in fact I did not have cancer at all.

The results were far from being fine – I was told that there were cancer cells still left in my breast after the lumpectomy and that I was being advised to have a mastectomy, followed by radiotherapy, chemotherapy and tamoxifen tablets. This sent me reeling into a black hole. For the first time in my life I felt so very hopeless and helpless. I just did not know what to do. Just the word cancer has so much stigma attached to it that it fills you with fear – in my shocked state it all felt so final.

The magic in this story really started about eight months before, however, in June 1996. I was having a rare and treasured lie-in when I started to daydream and from somewhere came the idea of power-walking the New York Marathon for charity – of course nobody would bat an eyelid to see power-walkers in a runners' road race, but if we were to wear decorated Wonderbras and get personalities and celebrities to endorse us, then that would be something else!

I literally jumped out of bed with this totally crazy idea and set about press-ganging a few friends. Looking back now, I realize just how bizarre it was, I knew nothing about marathons, power-walking and fundraising, and I certainly knew nothing about breast cancer – our chosen charity. I had to telephone Talking Pages to find the telephone number of a breast cancer charity – Breakthrough Breast Cancer was the one I was given.

After New York came the London Marathon, and Breakthrough had some places that we could use. I had no idea that within a few short weeks of my return from New York my own life would change beyond belief – that I would be diagnosed with breast cancer myself.

I was due to have my mastectomy eight weeks before the London Marathon and I did wonder if I would be able to take part. I so wanted to join the girls – sadly I would be walking in my T-shirt.

As strange as it may seem, I somehow managed to deal with the cancer in my mind, but found it impossible to come to terms with the thought of waking up with only one breast. Maybe spending so many years around models and body images had worn deeper than I thought or, maybe, just being quite young and single, it felt as though my life as a normal woman was over. I could not imagine that I would ever feel physically attractive again.

Two days before my operation I felt no more prepared to lose my breast than I ever had. Having had second opinions, and grilled my surgeon on whether there was another route to take, or if he had made a mistake, I always came back to the same distressing answer.

It was at this time that I had the good fortune of meeting with Rosy Daniel at the Bristol Cancer Centre. She was so supportive of my feelings and concerns, and she also recognized that I was still in a state of shock and recommended that I try to delay my operation. This was something that I had not even considered was possible – time had always seemed to be of the essence. The next day, just 24 hours before my surgery was due to take place, I spoke to my surgeon and asked him if it was possible to delay everything. Through the course of discussion he agreed. It was decided that he would delay my surgery by eight weeks if I promised to come back and if I felt that I could deal with it mentally. I felt as though I had been walked to the gallows and then just offered an eight-week reprieve. I felt very comfortable with the plan, but for a few people who were close to me it proved to be a very controversial decision. But I had to stand firm,

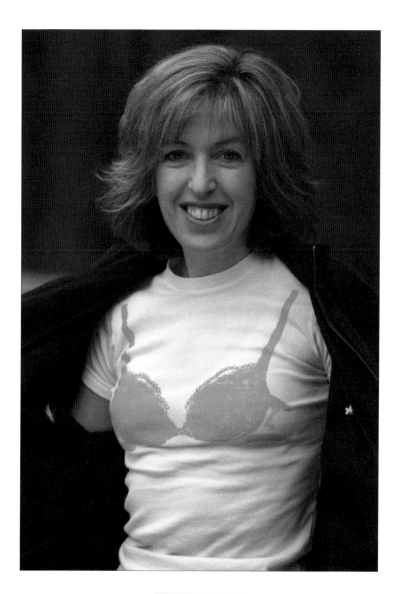

Nina Barough

and so I let go of a few more friends, for the time being anyway.

Meanwhile, the power-walking team were hard into training, bras were being signed by a host of people including the Spice Girls, Gary Lineker, Rod Stewart, Britt Ekland and Linda McCartney. My phone never stopped ringing with the girls telling me of their training stories or their fundraising conquests, and now with my new lease of life I was out there joining them, walking along to my affirmations of good health, great doctors and a normal life.

Eight weeks could have been eight years.

By the time the marathon came around, I certainly felt very fit and healthy. Each day had become a complete focus on what I ate and how I trained. In a funny way, I suppose I was leading the life of an athlete; I was certainly beginning to feel like one. If only my PE teacher from school could see me now! We also started to get a lot of publicity. Breakthrough asked me if I would share publicly my experience of breast cancer. At first I said no, I was not sure that I could face the exposure on something that was so fragile within me. People normally talk about their experiences after, not while it is still happening, and I did not know what the outcome would be. But as interviews for TV, radio and newspapers became more frequent, and the usual question of why are you doing this was asked, I realized I was being given an opportunity to share something very special. If I could talk about what was happening to me and if in turn it made a difference to even one person, then it somehow gave my situation some purpose. Through this I have learned that secrecy and fear are cancer's biggest allies. Each time I openly spoke about my treatment it felt wonderful, as though I was releasing a little of it, but even more importantly it allowed people to feel comfortable with me, and consequently the support I received from all sorts of places was like a big feather duvet wrapping itself around me.

The marathon was just tremendous, not to mention our grand finish walking down the Mall – 25 girls hand in hand, with an escort of motorbikes behind. Two days after the marathon we held the first Walk the Walk auction of bras and a photographic exhibition from our first walk in New York. What a night to remember! We sold our bras for £13,000, the champagne flowed and, despite our aching legs and sore feet, we were all flying on a magic carpet – with medals, of course! And of course the talk began about the possibility of doing the next New York Marathon the following November!

Just one week later, I was in hospital on the eve of my mastectomy, my reprieve over. I felt very well and I also felt a lot calmer and more prepared to face the ordeal. I had done everything that I had set out to do in the past eight weeks and now I could only trust in God, the universe, whatever you want to call the energy that supports us all. On 23 April, not only did St George fight his dragon, but I fought mine. I am happy to tell you that all the cancer cells were removed along with my breast. My biggest wish was that I could have a reconstruction at the same time. It is not always possible, but I got my wish.

Today as I sit and write this, Walk the Walk is about to make another quantum leap: the third Moonwalk, our own marathon which also started as an accident, will take place in May, and we already have over 3,000 entrants who will be starting their marathon at midnight, power-walking through the streets of London in their bras. This year will be our fifth New York Marathon, we have walked the Great Wall of China, taken part in the Beijing Marathon, the Dublin women's 10K, the Flora 3-mile challenge and the Great North Run, and everywhere we go we receive the most tremendous support. We truly are an ever-growing team of women.

It is my wish that one day there will be thousands of women walking the walk in a host of countries. I certainly have lots of ideas and plans for the future. It was never my intention to become a fundraiser, or to start a charity, so who knows how far it will go?

As for me, many magical things have happened over the past three years. Fitness and health are still major issues in my life, and I take part in all the Walk the Walk events. When you feel good, everything in life seems so much easier. I still have regular checks with my surgeon and so far so good.

As I write this it is almost 23 April again and I always make a point of celebrating. My big challenge at the moment is to feel comfortable being naked in front of other people such as in the gym changing rooms. I am not there yet but I am working on it.

I have the best friends and family – the support that they have given and do give me has allowed me to make this journey on my magic carpet. I have a very special man in my life, he helps me to keep my boots on the ground, the stress out of my shoulders and a big smile on my face. I have changed, I think for the better, certainly my focus on life has changed. Family and friends are the most important thing to me – they cannot be put on hold. I try to remember that each and every day is important – not always that easy in our society of forward planning. If I forget I only have to get undressed.

In fairy stories there is usually a happy ending. Well I can't tell you what's going to be, nobody can, but one very important lesson I have learned is to trust in the universe and it will always support you. I have put it to the test so I know it is true. Recently I came across part of a poem that really says everything for me:

Yesterday is history,
Tomorrow is a mystery
Today is a gift,
That is why it is called the present.

Me! – I love presents.

Nina's tips for surviving treatment

- Ask lots of questions and get a second opinion.

Nina's book recommendations

- *The Alchemist* by Paolo Coelho
- *Guarding the Three Treasures: The Chinese Way of Health* by Daniel Reid
- Also meditation tapes by Living Magically

Dedicated to my family, my friends and all the girls who have had the fun and courage to walk the walk and help me to conquer my dragon

BARBARA ELLIOTT

As sure as what is most sure, sure as that spring primroses
Shall new-dapple next year, sure as tomorrow morning,
Amongst come-back-again things, things with a revival, things with a
   recovery.

'AS SURE AS WHAT IS MOST SURE', GERARD MANLEY HOPKINS

Barbara Elliott, 45, lives with her partner Paul and their children, Emily, 21, and Thomas, 9, in Beccles, Suffolk. She has just received a First Class Honours degree from the University of East Anglia and hopes to study for her MA in Medical Anthropology, researching into illnesses such as breast cancer.

Barbara was diagnosed with breast cancer in 1994, aged 39. She completed nine months of chemotherapy and four weeks of radiotherapy, followed by a mastectomy at the James Paget Hospital, Suffolk.

Barbara's Story

I was 39. I had two children aged 16 and four. I had just applied to university to do a degree. And then I was diagnosed with breast cancer.

The diagnosis took about six weeks from my first going to my GP to the final pronouncement from the consultant at the hospital. This period of uncertainty and fear was far worse than knowing the diagnosis. Those six weeks took place over December and January and, in my memory, they have a grey and draining atmosphere, punctuated by Christmas Eve, Christmas Day and New Year. Those days were poignant, but at the same time I felt a growing determination that, whatever the results of the hospital tests, I was not going to become a victim of circumstance.

This attitude has been central to my experience of breast cancer. Although I felt that my body had let me down, I was still going to make the most of what I had – my family, my friends, my life. Also pivotal was the development of a seriously black humour, where cancer became the source of irony, and where unwanted sympathy – usually from people I hardly knew – was turned into a family joke.

During my nine months of chemotherapy and month of radiotherapy, I had an interview at the University of East Anglia. I told them nothing about the breast cancer, but instead persuaded them that, even though I had written nothing of any length for twenty years, I would be a dedicated student. They sent me off to write an essay about Bridget Riley, the abstract painter. Writing the essay was like getting blood out of a stone, but I finally succeeded, between bouts of chemotherapy, and was offered a place.

When the end of chemotherapy approached, I began to feel anxious. What would happen to me afterwards? At least during the months of treatment I felt safe, protected by the fact that I was under the wing of the hospital.

Three weeks after all my treatment had finished, I started at the university. It felt very strange. I'd swapped an institution I knew, that looked after me, for another which seemed alien and otherworldly. It was also full of people half my age.

At the end of my first year, the tumour in my breast returned. This was very frightening. I had to have a liver scan, a bone scan, and blood tests to check that the cancer hadn't spread. It hadn't. So I checked into the hospital to have a mastectomy.

After a week I left hospital and eight weeks later I went on holiday to the Cairngorms, walking and cycling. I would have tabloid headlines running through my mind – 'WOMAN WITH MASTECTOMY CLIMBS MOUNTAIN' . . . 'WOMAN WITH MASTECTOMY CYCLES THROUGH WILDERNESS'.

The surgery fitted neatly into the summer holiday and I returned in September to continue with my second year. I've nearly finished my degree – it has taken five years part time – and I feel very proud of myself: 'WOMAN WITH FOUR O-LEVELS AND MASTECTOMY AWARDED DEGREE'.

Although I define myself as a woman who has had a mastectomy, it is in the past. The scar represents a past event.

However, this event does not lose its potency – the memory and pain of cancer will always remain.

I realize that we all have to die, but I am not ready yet. Life is for experience and thinking and feeling. It's important to allow yourself to express your feelings about cancer, while making the most of ordinary things – cooking, eating, sunny days, rainy days, shopping. We need to feel as well as think. Allowing yourself to feel afraid or angry is not negative, it is positive. It is being real to yourself, so that you can get on with being happy. Feelings need to be felt.

When I had breast cancer, I used to go out in the car and shout. I used to go for bicycle rides and cry. I've been round our local supermarket crying. I feel this was a real achievement because I wasn't pretending that I felt OK when I didn't.

Cancer is a double-edged sword. It is awful, destructive, truly malignant. But it doesn't always kill you. It sharpens the mind and brings everything into focus. The possibility of a shortened future intensifies the present. We are forced to realize that we do only live once. This revelation can be a chance for re-evaluation. So find the people and places that make you feel good. I want to enjoy the company of my friends and family more. Do I want this job for the rest of my life? How can my presence in the world become a more positive force?

This has led me to two related but different activities. I joined a support group at the James Paget Hospital where I received my treatment. The group is made up of women who have all had some form of breast cancer. We attend clinics at the hospital, giving visible evidence that there is life after breast cancer, and give encourage-ment to women newly dealing with breast cancer.

My partner Paul has cycled 600 miles to raise money for Breakthrough. This cycle ride, my support group and this book all turn cancer into a positive force. By raising money for research into breast cancer my experience has turned into something positive for the future. For a long time I could not bear to think ahead beyond my next hospital check-up. But now I think further ahead. I am applying to do an MA. I am going to Los Angeles in the summer. Life *is* exciting and full of possibilities. Do the things you fancy doing. Don't be afraid to

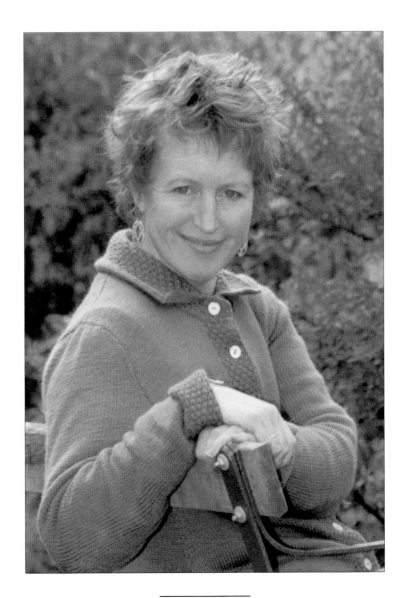

Barbara Elliott

cry, but don't forget to laugh. Enjoy yourself! 'WOMAN WITH MASTECTOMY LIVES. WOMAN WITH MASTECTOMY ENJOYS HERSELF!'

Barbara's tip for surviving treatment

- All types of therapy – retail therapy, taste-bud therapy, corny-film therapy, laughter therapy

Barbara's book recommendation

- Any informational literature from the Bristol Cancer Help Centre (see Cancer Support Addresses)

Dedicated to my family and friends

PAULINE SILVERMAN

Cancer changes your life for ever – change it around and make something good happen out of something which could have been so bad.

Pauline Silverman, 50, is Personnel Manager for a kitchen wholesale and distribution company. She lives in Abbots Langley, Hertfordshire, with her two cats, Jaspa and Kara. She has a son, Spencer, 26, and a daughter, Gayle, 24.

Pauline was diagnosed with breast cancer in 1991, aged 41. She had a partial mastectomy at the BUPA Hospital, Bushey, followed by five weeks of radiotherapy at the Mount Vernon Hospital, Northwood, Middlesex, and six years of tamoxifen.

Pauline's Story

As I stood at the top of Striding Edge, taking in the awesome panoramic view of the sun-drenched Lake District below me, I reflected that it was three times a miracle that I was there. Firstly, a miracle because I get vertigo standing on a kitchen stool. Secondly, a miracle that in the past ten days I had walked some 150 miles from Robin Hood's Bay in North Yorkshire when previously the furthest distance I had walked was from John Lewis to Fenwick's at Brent Cross. But the most amazing miracle was that I was alive and fit to do this coast-to-coast walk for Breakthrough since it was only twelve months before this that I was diagnosed with that life-threatening disease that send shivers of fear through any woman – breast cancer.

I remembered my first consultation with the specialist. I already knew him because his children had attended the same school as mine. We were catching up on the news of their progress so it seemed more like a social event than anything else. Perhaps that's why I sat there numbed and struck dumb when he told me that the mammogram had shown a lesion in the right breast highly suggestive of a carcinoma.

I remember that he said he needed to do a biopsy and that this would probably be followed by a partial mastectomy if the pathology report came back indicating malignancy. He said that this should be arranged as soon as possible. Fortunately, as I had private medical insurance through my employers, we managed to get the ball rolling and one week later I was waking up from the anaesthetic, being told the bad news.

It was incredible how the lump was discovered in the first place. I had been getting sharp shooting pains behind the left nipple but I took no notice for a couple of weeks and thought it might be indigestion or a heart attack or that my bra was too tight. It was Gayle who nagged me to see a doctor as she was embarrassed to be seen with me in Sainsbury's breaking out in a cold sweat, doubled over with pain and hanging on to my left breast.

The GP sent me for a chest X-ray, an ECG and a mammogram and when I went to see him a couple of days later for the result, he had that 'I've got some worrying news for you' look on his face. The strange thing was that the lump was deep in the right breast, and the fact that pains in my left breast had sent me to see him in the first place made me think that someone up there was watching over me. Had I not seen the doctor then, the lump would doubtless have grown and grown until it manifested itself on the surface and by then, who knows, it may have been too late!

The week between seeing the specialist and having the biopsy was the longest week of my life. Daytime wasn't too bad because I had my very hectic job to keep me occupied, and the evenings were bearable because I was busy keeping house and helping Spencer and Gayle with their homework. But once they had gone to bed, I was alone with my thoughts and fears. What do you do when you can't sleep at night, when you can't concentrate on television or reading or the radio and when it's an unsociable hour to call a friend? I cleaned the oven (not that it was dirty in the first place I'll have you know) and it's amazing how scrubbing and scrubbing and scrubbing vents your anger and relieves your tension. When I couldn't scrub the oven any

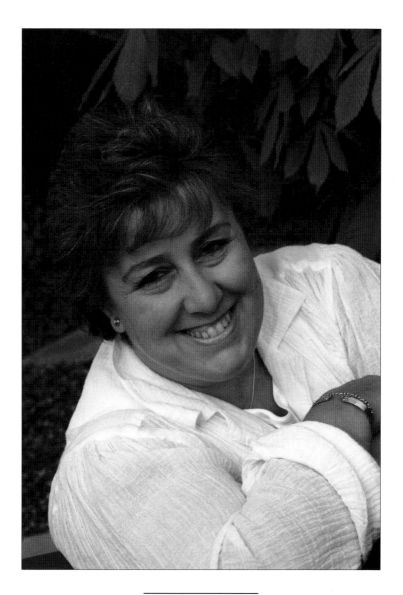

Pauline Silverman

more for fear of wearing away the walls, I cleaned the windows. You'd be amazed how therapeutic it is to clean windows in the dark. You can't see whether or not they're clean, so you do it again and again. The only downside is that if my neighbours had seen me cleaning the windows in the dark at 3 a.m., it would have confirmed their suspicions about me!

I didn't really talk to the kids too much about it because I didn't want to frighten them. They knew I had to go into hospital for investigations but I didn't want to mention the word cancer until I had to. So when it was confirmed, we talked about it and they were pretty good. Fortunately, while I was in hospital, I was looking and feeling well, so thank goodness they didn't see me as a 'sick' person. Once the radiotherapy started, some four weeks after the surgery, again I was fortunate that I kept well. Other than intermittent tiredness and some nausea, you couldn't tell that I was having treatment. My boss allowed me to work in the mornings (I was anxious to get back to work just to keep things as normal as possible), and in the afternoons an array of friends would taxi me to and from Mount Vernon Hospital. Sometimes I would come home feeling fine and it would just be a normal day for me and the kids, but sometimes I was that tired that I just had to go to bed.

Jaspa and Kara, my ever faithful pussycats, were wonderful company and certainly contributed towards my recovery. Lying in bed or sitting on the settee with a warm purring cat on your lap is incredibly relaxing and therapeutic. Much more so than scrubbing the oven, which I couldn't do anyway because of the restricted movement in my arm.

At the end of the five weeks of continual radiotherapy, I was keen to just get on with my life. However, my life had changed. I'd been faced with a life-threatening disease. I fleetingly considered the possibility that I wouldn't see my children grow up. Spencer was 15, Gayle 13, and we had survived some difficult times following my divorce so I was blowed if this was going to get the better of me. I wanted to channel my energies and turn the situation around by making something good happen out of what could have been (and still could be) so terrible.

My saviour was Breakthrough Breast Cancer, a new charity. I had read that they were looking for 15,000 challengers to each raise at least £1,000 to help fund the £15 million needed to establish a new research centre totally dedicated to breast cancer. I asked my boss, Stuart, if the company would be willing to support me in my fundraising activities and he gladly agreed. I was not the first person within our organization to be affected by breast cancer, so the cause was dear to his heart as well as mine. So, in October 1991, seven months after my diagnosis, I began planning an adventure which would change my life, and in August 1992, there I was standing at the top of Striding Edge reflecting on all this. That was just the beginning.

One year later I was sitting next to my faithful friend Rochelle on our side-by-side recumbent tricycle at John O'Groats, in the rain, ready to cycle 1,000 miles to Land's End. Two and a half weeks later, after a most amazing adventure, we arrived in Land's End, exhausted but sun-tanned (or was it rust), heavier rather than slimmer after all those wonderful Scottish breakfasts but, more than anything, overwhelmed by the generosity of all those who had supported us along the way.

There were so many people in the Breakthrough network of supporters who arranged local fundraising events around our visit to their area and opened their homes to feed and water us and wash our smalls (or rather our bigs) and provide us with somewhere to rest our weary heads at night. There were so many funny incidents – I wish I had the room to tell you about crossing the Forth Road Bridge, or tea with the Mayor of Hereford in his parlour, or the horse at the bottom of the hill. Well, maybe another time in another book! There were also those people who stopped us on the road to ask what we were doing and to put money in the collection tins. I can't tell you how many people stopped to take photographs of us – why would they want our double chins in their photo album?

These fundraising adventures were extremely rewarding but unbelievably tiring, so now I tend to do things like put on concerts (my passion is singing) to raise funds. But the cycle is sitting in Rochelle's garage eagerly awaiting its next outing. We've taken it over to the

European mainland on other adventures, again another story for another time.

Now, nine years after diagnosis, I am still eagerly working to help fund research. Unfortunately, my family has a terrible breast cancer track record with three of my mother's sisters and three daughters in my generation being affected. Some of us had the genes test, but thank goodness it appears to be 'clustering', rather than the faulty gene. To all you who are reading this book, be positive. Breast cancer is a terrible thing but there is life and hope during and afterwards. Cancer changes your life, but it can and often is for the better. Make something good happen out of it. I wish you well.

Pauline's tips for surviving treatment

- Be positive.
- Take one day at a time and don't panic.
- Get as much rest as possible but do things to keep your mind occupied. Remember, everybody has different reactions to the treatment and it certainly isn't always horrendous. I was able to continue working all through my period of radiotherapy treatment and I met people who were working through periods of chemotherapy.

Pauline's book recommendation

- *Breakthrough into Verse: A Book of Poems* by Jenny Whiteside (with proceeds to go to Breakthrough Breast Cancer)

Pauline's music recommendation

- Vivaldi's *Four Seasons*

Dedicated to Spencer and Gayle, my family and friends, Jaspa and Kara (my pussycats!)

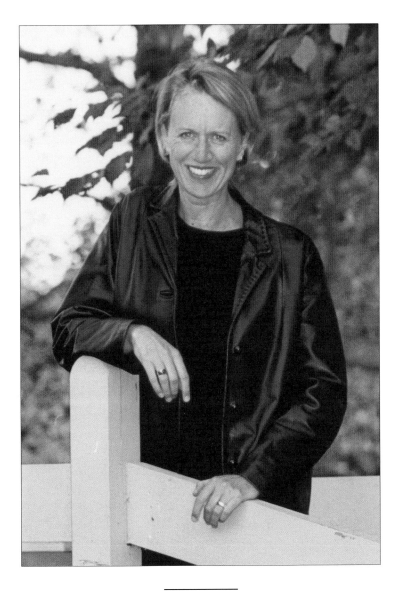

Sally Taylor

SALLY TAYLOR

Laughter is the best medicine.

Sally Taylor, 45, is a broadcaster and journalist and presents BBC South's nightly news magazine programme, *South Today*. She lives with her partner John Paul in Winchester.

Sally was diagnosed with breast cancer in 1999, aged 43, at Sarum Road Hospital, Winchester. She had DCIS (ductal carcinoma *in situ*) in her right breast but opted for a bilateral mastectomy with *Latissimus dorsi* reconstruction.

Sally's Story

My mother died from breast cancer when I was six years old. It was 1961 and I still have her letters describing her long and tiring weekly trips to the hospital by bus, train and then ambulance for her treatment.

In March 1999, I was diagnosed with DCIS which was the very early stages of cancer in my right breast. Maybe with my family history I shouldn't have been surprised but I was shocked when I was told I needed a mastectomy.

I had assumed that because the cancer was caught so early I would be put on a drug treatment programme. I was completely unprepared for the traumatic news. It happened on the day I was presenting a quiz on *Noel's House Party*. To this day I have no idea what I said or did, my mind was somewhere else. I was numb. Talk about from the sublime to the ridiculous!

After learning that there was a slight chance of developing it in my left breast, I opted to have the other breast removed as well . . . many people have said that was a brave decision to take, but for me it was obvious because it was a huge relief to eradicate the problem. All this happened as I began a new relationship with a lovely man . . . I had only met John Paul three months before and although we were committed to each other, this was to be one of the biggest tests of our relationship. He was fantastic, always there and always supportive in so many ways. He helped me to face my fears and overcome them. It's brought us much closer together. I feel very lucky to have met him.

As a journalist I have a naturally enquiring mind so it was important for me to read anything and everything about the ordeal I faced. By reading, asking questions and meeting other women who had been through similar experiences, I felt that I was empowering myself. Without doubt, the whole episode was less traumatic because I knew what was going to happen, good and bad. A good piece of advice is: make sure your surgeon and doctor answer your questions but bear in mind that when you first hear the news, you will be absolutely shell-shocked and you'll sit there not thinking of a single question to ask. But once you've had time to absorb the news, make a list of things you want to know; it doesn't matter how simple or ridiculous the question, *ask* it. Your surgeon should answer it, certainly mine did.

One of the brilliant schemes that Winchester Hospital runs is for women who are facing major surgery for breast cancer to meet those who've already been through the ordeal. We nicknamed it 'Bosom Buddies'! And for me it was a major turning point. I had been so afraid of the operation; I wasn't sure if I would still look good. Would my breasts look natural again? Would my man still want me and what about sex – would it still be exciting and passionate? Or would I look and feel like a freak? Meeting these women was inspiring . . . they were living their lives to the full, they looked great and they bared all to show me!

I came away without any doubts about the operation I was facing. Yes it was a major op, ten hours long, to remove both breasts and reconstruct new ones using muscles from my back and bags full of saline solution. It's become known as the scarless mastectomy and it looks great – or rather *they* look great!

Before my op there was so much to sort out; not only did I need to get my life in order but there was the inevitable question whether I should go public or keep it a secret. I'd been presenting the BBC's *South Today* for twelve years so if I had taken four months off without any explanation there would have been a lot of speculation. Anyway, I've always felt that keeping a secret is a burden in itself.

Thank goodness I had a great boss who allowed me to set the pace. JP and I could decide when we were ready to tell everyone and then the huge BBC machine went into action. I had no idea the effect this announcement would have but I was inundated with good wishes, flowers and support from so many people. I was totally overwhelmed!

One of the first things that struck me was just how many people are touched by cancer. It seemed that almost everyone had a story and most of them were uplifting and optimistic. It's so easy to feel the worst when you're facing cancer and, of course, it's often the negative side of statistics you hear. But when you share your fears with others and discover there are so many other people who are living with cancer, it helps to put your own worries into context . . . you are not alone. And there are so many positive and encouraging testimonies.

I have always had a wicked sense of humour and somehow I held on to that throughout this difficult time. I'll admit there were lots of tears as well but even that is part of the healing process. Don't keep things bottled up. I had decided I needed to have breast recon-struction at the same time as my mastectomy. I had a new and important relationship and I was still young. I didn't think I would feel confident about my body and myself without reconstruction.

Every cloud has a silver lining! I could choose the size of my new breasts! One of the ladies I had met had always desired large breasts so she had gone from a 34B to a 36DD and she looked great. So when my surgeon asked me I just laughed and said I had no idea. 'Think about it,' he said. So John Paul and I used this opportunity to leaf through those magazines you only ever find on the top shelf of newsagents'! When the time came we went back to our surgeon and showed him the pair we fancied!! All I need to tell you is that I'm happy, John Paul is happy and, to be truthful, they're almost the same size as before.

I won't deny it was a difficult period of my life and equally difficult for my partner. But now I'm out on the other side and I can look back and I feel as though I've changed. It's true your priorities do alter. Things that you have taken for granted before become very important. I felt as though I had been emptied of everything, no energy and no emotion left. It gave me the opportunity to spend time to look at my life and see if it was all I wanted. I came to the conclusion I needed to change. It was a rebuilding exercise, everything had been stripped out and the foundations were laid to start all over again.

So has my life changed for the better? Yes, I think it has, even though sometimes my priorities revert back to what they were before my operation. It's so easy to knock things down but it takes much longer to build things back up. It takes time and patience, and confidence in yourself that it can be done.

Facing breast cancer is difficult but each one of us has an inner strength and it's during these difficult times that we find it. So don't be afraid, face the problem with confidence and be positive but never be afraid to cry – I promise you it does help!

Sally's tips for surviving treatment

- ❀ Stay positive.
- ❀ Keep asking questions of your surgeon and his or her team.

Sally's book recommendations

- ❀ Books by Carl Hiaasen: *Lucky You*; *Stormy Weather*; *Double Whammy*; *Strip Tease*; *Skin Tight*; *Kiss Ass: Selected Columns*, among others

Dedicated to my mother Dorothy Taylor who died of breast cancer when she was in her thirties and I was just six years old

SHARON MADDRELL

Cancer? Been there, done that, got the T-shirt!

Sharon Maddrell, 48, is manager of the Ramsey Post Office on the Isle of Man. With four other breast cancer patients she has started the only support group on the island. She has learned to ski, abseil, parapent and keep her sense of humour.

Sharon was diagnosed with breast cancer, a Stage II ductal carcinoma, in 1995, aged 43. She had a lumpectomy at Nobles Hospital, Isle of Man, followed by five weeks of radiotherapy at Clatterbridge Hospital, Wirral.

Sharon's Story

31 January 1995

Went for the mammogram and needle aspiration on my own, as I thought everything was OK. Saw the pathologist after the mammogram. He was really nice. He did the job and went off to test it and I sat chatting with the nurse. He returned . . . 'I'm sorry. There's no easy way of saying this, but . . .' I wasn't expecting it and just wept.

I left the hospital and went to my cousin Judy's. She was waiting for me. I told her and we cried together. She came with me to tell Mum. It was hard after Dad dying three years ago from cancer. It must have seemed very cruel to her, first him, now me. She appeared to take it very well, at least while we were with her. I asked Judy to ring around my friends. Mum rang my brother in Chester. I talked to him. He was lovely and quite determined I would be all right – so I will! He'd be too angry if I wasn't.

2 February

My appointment with the surgeon Mr Lee. Judy came with me. I went in on my own. The lovely nurse just asked me how I'm coping, and I burst into tears! Mr Lee examined me and decided that all that was needed was a lumpectomy at Nobles Hospital, Isle of Man, and a trip to Clatterbridge Hospital Oncology Unit in Wirral. Tears of relief. He will arrange for me to come into hospital when I'm back from skiing.

4 February

Off to Austria for the best holiday I've ever had and the biggest laugh. Somehow I didn't think about it at all. Ain't life strange? I was kept so busy skiing, drinking and laughing, there really wasn't time!! From Manchester Airport I rang up my friend Bernice, to see when I go into hospital and it's Thursday. There's one thing about all this, they don't hang about.

17 February

Operation at 10.30 a.m. Came to about 1.00 p.m. to hear my friend Netty's voice outside. Am I ready for this? Yes I am. I feel absolutely fine. She had me in tears laughing in two minutes – she thought the drain from my boob was a catheter! I did a quick check that they had only taken the lump and was relieved to see that they had.

I'm getting out tomorrow at 12.00 noon to go shopping with Mum.

23 February

My appointment with the famous Dr Hughes, the Clatterbridge oncologist. I have Stage II cancer in the milk duct and need 20 treatments of radiotherapy.

I rang Debbie, my friend in Canada, who has had breast cancer three times, to tell her the news. She has been great, having gone through a lot worse herself. We have talked often (ouch – the phone bill) about how we feel and how to cope. I think I'm doing OK. I see a lot of my dad in me thankfully – the wish to get on with the treatment, get it over with without too much disruption and fuss. I can't have this interrupting my social life! Fortunately, it doesn't.

Through all this, I haven't once thought, 'Why me?' Why not me? Cancer is totally indiscriminate. It will get whoever it can lay its grubby hands on. I believe our lives are predestined anyway, there's nothing we can do to change the course of things, so you may as well accept what life throws at you and get on with it the best you can!

3 March

Got the most awful flu and felt so rough. Isn't it funny how you feel so bad with flu, yet somebody tells you you've got cancer and you feel so bloody healthy! How do they do that?

7 March

My birthday, and my brother Kerry came with me to Clatterbridge Hospital for the start of my radiotherapy. Kerry is such a lovely man and I am so proud of him. Maybe I'll tell him how much I love him one day. After a bottle of red!

Saw Dr Hughes, the oncologist, and had my planning done. Lots of purple lines and crosses on my boob. Treatment starts tomorrow.

8 March

First treatment. It's nothing. Strip off, lie down, don't move, zap zap, bye-bye, two mins! Life is like a rollercoaster ride at present. One minute you're up there, next it's 'Oh shit', down you go.

I went home for the weekend as it was Mother's Day. Mum didn't know so it was a nice surprise for her. I am still feeling fine.

The treatment is being very kind to me. I have no effects except a slight reddening of the skin like mild sunburn. However, I'd kill for a shower! I do hate not doing any exercise and I'm eating like a horse. My sister-in-law Mavis's great cooking, and eating out – it's a hard life.

6 April

Last treatment. A strange feeling prevails that's hard to explain. The treatment's gone by so fast. I've had such a good time here. Spent more time with Kerry than I have since we were children. I really feel sad at leaving Clatterbridge for the last time, yet glad also, obviously. Perhaps it's because I'm on my own now. The whole thing has certainly not been an unpleasant experience, just an experience . . .

7 April

I left Kerry's. I wanted to say so much but didn't want to get soppy, so I left a couple of bottles of wine and a card thanking them. It would not have been half as easy without them.

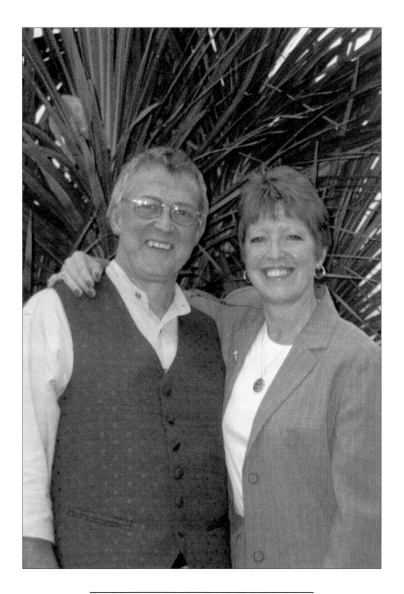

Sharon Maddrell with brother Kerry

It feels strange to be home for good. Mum is glad to see that I still look well and is glad to have me back. (She could worry for England!)

26 April

I feel great and want to put all this behind me and get on with life. I sometimes stop and think, 'Have I ever had cancer?' It doesn't feel like I have as I have been so lucky and the treatment did not trouble me at all really. Still a bit tired and I am off work until 15 May. I've noticed over the last couple of weeks that the colour has gone from my nipple! The only visible effect of the radiotherapy. It looks funny. Still, it could be an ice-breaker at parties!

28 August 1999

Appointment with the oncologist for my yearly check-up. He sent me for a mammogram – two years since my last one. Nerves frazzled again! I rang up for the results (couldn't wait!) – it's clear!

Almost five years on now, no medication (just been taken off tamoxifen). No lasting effects unless you count no hair in the armpit that received radiotherapy (killed off the hair follicles); anyway saves on the Immac!

My priorities in life have completely changed, I don't take anything for granted. I never say I'm cured. If someone asks if I'm all clear I just say, 'Hopefully.'

Sharon's tips for surviving treatment

- Try and contact someone who's been through it.
- Plan a holiday for when the treatment's over.
- Don't look back in anger; only look forward to life and enjoy it.

Sharon's book recommendation

- *Laughter Is the Best Therapy* by Robert Holden.

Dedicated to my dad Jack who died of cancer in 1992. I'm glad he didn't have to watch me go through it, but seeing how brave he was inspired me when my turn came.

OLIVIA NEWTON-JOHN

My memories are inside me – they're not things or a place – I can take them anywhere.

Olivia Newton-John, 51, is a well-known actress/singer who lives in Malibu, California, with her daughter Chloe, 14. She is best known for her starring roles in the films *Grease* and *Xanadu*, as well as her record career, including one of her bestselling singles, 'Let's Get Physical'.

Olivia was diagnosed with breast cancer in 1992, aged 44, in Los Angeles. She had a partial mastectomy with immediate reconstruction, followed by eight months of chemotherapy. She is currently eight years clear of any cancer and has never felt stronger physically and spiritually.

Olivia's Story

They say that divorce, bereavement, illness and moving house are the most traumatic things to deal with in life and I faced them all in three years. The cancer and bereavement were devastating but probably the hardest of all to face was divorce.

Slowly I have rebuilt my life. I went to a therapist the day after being diagnosed with cancer because a friend said I needed to talk to someone, an outsider, to get this out, although it was not something I had contemplated before. The way I was brought up in England and Australia, people thought you had to be really mentally sick to go into therapy, but I have learned from living in the US that there is a different attitude. If you have a broken tooth you go to the dentist. If you have emotional problems you see a therapist. It has helped me. I am not embarrassed to say it. I don't feel I have failed now. I feel fine. I'm fit and healthy. I've passed the critical five-year point with the cancer and now I only have to go for yearly checks.

Life is wonderful and I'm enjoying the freedom of being single.

When you have a child you never feel alone. Chloe, my daughter, is such a great companion.

I learned about my breast cancer the day after my dad died. I was with Matt (my ex-husband) and some friends on the San Juan Islands off the west coast of America for the Fourth of July weekend when the news came that my father had died. We were getting a seaplane to Seattle when Matt took a phone call. Apparently, there were two messages: one from my doctor saying he needed to see me and another telling me about my dad. Matt decided to save the news about the doctor until after the weekend. He thought Dad's death was enough for me to contend with.

We were sitting in a spot overlooking the sea at sunset; there was a bunch of friends with us. We drank a toast to Dad because all my friends loved him. I did not have much time to grieve because a day later I had the news about my cancer. My reaction was almost to laugh – like, what more can happen? What's going on here? There must be a reason. It did cross my mind that this was my pay-back for the good times. But I never felt angry or thought that it wasn't fair. Other people felt that for me but I never did. If anything, I came to see it as a challenge. I had to make a decision then. I had to decide: 'Do I go along with this or do I really fight it?'

The human mind is very strong and very powerful. I knew in my heart that my thoughts would affect my outcome and that I had to think positively to heal. I often used visualization of my beloved dog running through my veins eating up my cancer cells! This may sound odd but the more you can personalize your visualizations, the better they will work. Obviously, there would be moments. I'd be lying if I said there weren't moments, but I decided I was fine.

Just after I finished my treatment, I wrote and produced a very personal album called *Gaia*. One of my songs is called 'Why Me?' When something happens people often say, 'Why me, what have I done to deserve this?' But they shouldn't say, 'Why me?' They should say, 'Why not me?' Because often things happen for a reason. I really believe this happened to me for a reason.

I have always been very healthy: a vegetarian for a long time, I never drink, never smoke, I've never taken drugs, I've always

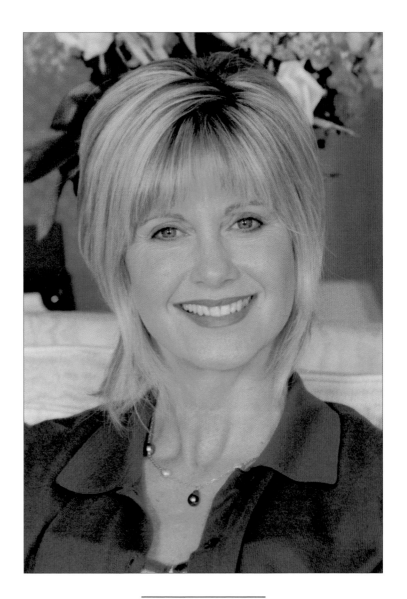

Olivia Newton-John

exercised – all these things. But I had been under a lot of stress and I was trying to take care of everybody. I tended to be a person who suppressed emotions, and if I was upset, I'd push it down. I wouldn't often let people know how I was feeling or if I was angry, because I had this good-girl, nice-girl image and I wasn't supposed to get angry. But it can be very unhealthy to push it down. The first thing the therapist asked me was: 'Have you been taking care of everyone?' And I said that I had and told her about my life. She said, 'You've been breast-feeding everybody. You've got to let them go – you've got to wean them off you.' It was a kind of revelation. It was a good image for me. The message was to take care of myself because I had always been putting everybody else before me. It's a bad thing we're taught in society, especially women, that taking care of yourself is a selfish thing. But it's really important to take care of yourself, because if you don't, you aren't able to take care of those around you. Women try hard to be everything to everybody and eventually something has to give. So I knew from that point I had to take care of myself.

Cancer is such a horrible word. Everybody associates it with death. But it is not necessarily a death sentence and many people do survive. I think the first couple of days, especially the first night, were the most frightening. I had a night of dread; I shall never forget it. I woke in the early hours with an overwhelming fear. I walked down to the kitchen and my body was so leaden I could hardly move. Then I made a decision. I said to myself, 'You're going to be OK,' and from that moment I fervently believed I would recover. I quickly made up my mind to be positive about it after my dearest friend who had been through it all herself told me, 'Your attitude is going to set the mood for everybody around you.' What scared me the most was the prospect of chemotherapy because I'm somebody who doesn't even like taking aspirin.

I feel very lucky that it was caught early and that it was not aggressive. I am fortunate because I was all right. I felt very supported throughout the treatment. Although I had chemotherapy, I didn't lose my hair, which was a psychological bonus. I wore an ice-cap – a sort of tea cosy filled with ice cubes – which is supposed to help. I looked very funny though. I looked like Mrs Mop!

I don't think I'm afraid of growing old any more, which is a wonderful release for me after going through my scare with breast cancer. I think it released me of all those fears and I think that was what it was all about: face life, face death, face illness; and now I think I can deal with almost anything. It sounds ironic to say that breast cancer is probably the best thing that happened to me, but really I think that in many ways it was. Facing death gives you a whole new view of life and helps you focus on the important things – like your family and your health. It made me grow up a lot, it made me work out my priorities and it made me let go of a lot of things that I didn't need to be doing and that I felt I had to be doing. It has, in retrospect, been a very positive experience.

Olivia's tips for surviving treatment

- To support myself I did homeopathy, herbs, acupuncture, yoga – everything I could to balance my system and be as strong as I could.
- I also meditated and prayed every single day. I covered all the bases.

Olivia's book recommendations

- All books by Louise Hay
- All books by Deepak Chopra

Dedicated to my daughter Chloe; Colette, my god-daughter; and my father Brinley Newton-John

Based on a series of interviews in the *Daily Mail* by Richard Shears (23 September 1994), Corinna Honan (25 January 1995) and Frances Hardy (23 May1998)

PATTIE COLDWELL

I may die from breast cancer. I may get run over by a bus. But it's not the dying that's the problem, but living and finding happiness in the struggle. So my death will not be tragic. It will be a celebration of my life.

Pattie Coldwell, 48, is a broadcaster and journalist. She lives in Berkshire. She has a daughter, Dannie, 8.

Pattie was diagnosed with breast cancer in 1997, aged 45, at the Royal Hampshire Hospital, Basingstoke. She had a lumpectomy followed by six months of chemotherapy at the Royal Hampshire Hospital and five weeks of radiotherapy in Southampton. Following a recurrence a year later, she had axillary clearance.

Pattie's Story

When I was diagnosed with breast cancer three summers ago, I was scared for about half an hour. The inevitable selfish question emerged as I cried in fear and confusion on my husband Tony's shoulder, outside the hospital – 'Why me?' My soul answered that question immediately. From deep down inside I felt I knew the reason I had developed cancer at the tender age of 45. Because I wasn't happy with myself. I was suppressing my real feelings, my real needs and wasting my dreams. I felt my feelings had literally cancered inside me.

To anyone who knows me, the idea that I suppress my feelings is ridiculous. As a broadcaster (and a human being!) I have established a reputation as outspoken, down-to-earth and searingly honest. I am emotional and passionate and appear to speak my mind at all times. But at that terrible moment, faced with my imminent death, I saw the truth. That I was covering my softer feelings. What I showed the world, and even my closest loved ones, was a tough, confident and, all too often, aggressive woman. The real, vulnerable and spiritual me had been covered for so long in the blustering pursuit

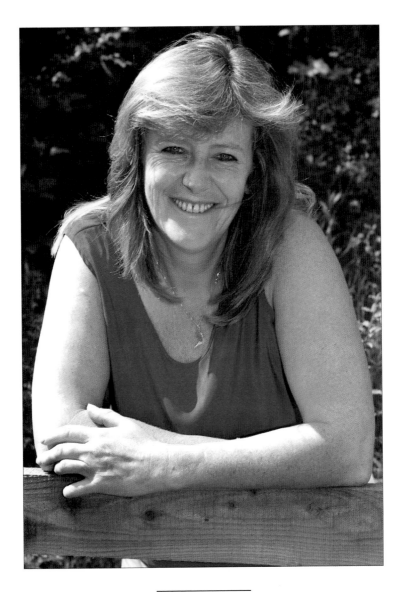

Pattie Coldwell

of love, career, fame and fortune. I realized in a flash that I had to change my life if I was to die happy.

On the face of it my life was as good as anyone could hope for. A handsome, loving husband, a lovely five-year-old daughter, devoted friends and family and a beautiful country home in five and a half acres of land. I was presenting three programmes, including Channel 5's new morning show with Tony, so the creative needs were also being fed and the money was pouring in too. But I felt my life was going nowhere. I couldn't seem to appreciate all I had. My sense of humour was on holiday and so was my sex life. I smoked and drank too much and worried all the time about what other people thought. I tried to help others but always ended up being interfering and bossy. I was stressed and, frankly, aimless. And now I had breast cancer.

But, as bad as the situation seemed, my new awareness gave me hope. There was something I could do, not to fight the cancer but to love it away. I had a purpose. Suddenly the fear disappeared and my new life began from there.

For the first few months, through chemotherapy, radiotherapy, losing my hair (and, on one charming occasion, my stomach lining), I was very proud of how I was coping. People called me brave for being so positive and, frankly, I agreed with them! I carried on working – at one point on all three programmes at the same time. Suddenly, I felt my life had a direction. I could now find my true self, which was generous, kind and optimistic. In my position as a broadcaster I could help other people to cope. And if I had to go all through this, it was a real opportunity to like myself! I had this feeling that one day I would actually be able to say I was glad I got cancer.

Tony stuck by me. He did everything he could possibly do to help when I was incapacitated. Looking after Dannie, most importantly, shopping, cleaning, organizing and running our big house. The first year was hard, but we seemed to be coming through. Then came the worst possible news – I had another lump under my arm. Surely this meant the cancer was travelling and it was only a matter of time before it killed me. We were all exhausted and very scared.

Incredibly, when the lump and my lymph nodes were removed, tests showed I was completely cancer-free. After an agonizing week of waiting, we rejoiced at my good fortune. Now, nearly two years on, there are still no signs of any more outbreaks. I am a very lucky lady. I have lost 40 pounds of the 50 I put on during the treatment, and I look and feel healthier than I have in many years. At 48 I've started to see the path to real happiness. There's just one problem. Tony doesn't share it with me.

We are now separated and getting a divorce. I wish I could tell you that everything is now fine, that I have come out the other end happier and calmer and that the cancer brought us closer. But it's not true . . . so far. As I write, we are arguing about where Dannie is going to live and there is a lot of bitterness and pain in the air. We are all suffering and trying to understand what's happened. Tony and I both have new partners and some of our friends and family have taken sides. So it's a very difficult time. My heart aches for what poor Dannie has had to cope with in her short little life and I grieve the loss of a relationship that I truly believed would go on for ever.

Bearing in mind that life has a way of slapping you in the face with a wet fish just as you think you're getting it together, how do you follow your dreams and find happiness when everything around seems bleak? Hey! If I knew the answer to that one I'd do it. But I can share what I'm learning through all this struggle. I'm beginning to forgive myself, learn from my mistakes and move forward one day at a time. A lot of me just wants to run away and escape but I'm hanging on in there. I lose my way regularly and fall into all the bad habits, but what helps me are optimism and faith and recognizing that I am only human. I have no god in my world, but I'm yearning for a more spiritual and simple life. So when things look bleak, I now try to focus on what's positive, on what I have and what is today.

Take this week. On the downside: I rowed with Tony and we said some terrible things that we didn't mean; Dannie didn't want to see me, I felt she didn't love me; I had far too much to drink, and took it out on someone very dear to me; I ate badly; I smoked too much; I didn't sleep enough; I complained at work. Oh yes, and I got grumpy with a swimming-pool attendant. But looked at in another way, focusing on the good things, it's a very different week indeed: Tony and I made friends again; Dannie was loving and caring the following day; my friend who got the angry verbals has forgiven me; I've been eating fruit and cutting down the drinking again; some dear friends are coming this weekend; and I've found a brilliant plumber to fit my central heating. I could go on about the blossom in my garden, my daughter's beautiful eyes, my lovely parents, the smell of cut grass and all the smaller things I now appreciate so much more, but let's not get too hippie about this!

The point is, it's one step at a time. Sometimes five forward and ten back, but I can feel it coming. I wasn't particularly scared of my cancer, so why should I be scared of my life? I've made some awful mistakes – but which of us hasn't? Time is too short not to learn from our mistakes. Let go and move forward. One day, I truly believe, Tony and I will be the closest of friends and the best of parents, even though we no longer live together. Those who have judged will understand and Dannie will be a happy, hearty young woman, who knows deep down that however mad her mum is, she tried her best and loved her. I want her to realize, as I have done, that you must love and respect yourself before you can truly love someone else. Change is always difficult, but if we have faith in our true feelings, anything is possible.

As my dear friend Terry Maidley said, when he was diagnosed with AIDS: 'I may die of AIDS. I may get run over by a bus. It's not the dying that's the problem, it's living and finding happiness in the struggle. So my death will not be tragic, it will be a celebration of my life.' Terry's funeral was a wonderful party and so will mine be. There will be many more struggles to come but I fully intend to be able to say on my deathbed, 'I'm glad I got breast cancer.'

Pattie's tips for surviving treatment

- Information is power so ask as many questions as possible.
- Take one step at a time.

Pattie's book recommendation

- *The Art of Happiness* by the Dalai Lama and Howard Cutler

Dedicated to my daughter Dannie, and to Tony

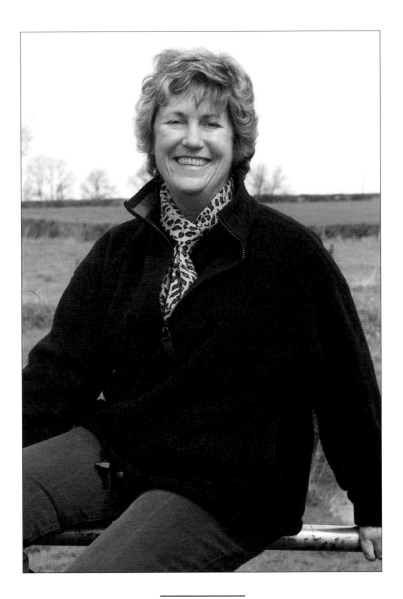

Pamela Hicks

PAMELA HICKS

Two roads diverged in a wood, and I –
I took the one less traveled by,
And that has made all the difference.
'THE ROAD NOT TAKEN', ROBERT FROST

Pamela Hicks, 58, is a retired teacher of English and drama. She lives with her husband John in England and France. She has two children, Rachel, 30, and Simon, 28.

Pamela was diagnosed with breast cancer in 1992, aged 50, at the John Radcliffe Churchill Hospital in Oxford. She had an invasive ductal carcinoma for which she received a lumpectomy at Horton Hospital, Banbury, and radiotherapy at the Churchill Hospital, Oxford.

Pamela's Story

What appals me is that I cannot actually remember the year my mother was diagnosed with cancer. I do know that the news came by phone. First, she told me a lump under her arm had to be checked. The next call, from my father, said that the lump was malignant.

My diary for June 1978 does record: 'Mum signed off treatment.' It refers to her chemotherapy. I really understood very little about cancer or the treatment. Less was written then and anyway I had no motivation to read it. Ignorance made me even more afraid for Mum. There seemed little I could say to her and less to my more nervous father. I am always more deeply affected by pain in others than in myself because I have no way of controlling their suffering.

Mum was in her sixties, Dad had recently retired. She was an attractive, educated woman, a practical and caring leader and someone who loved company. She was good company herself – she was Divisional Commissioner for Girl Guides and had danced and sung in amateur musicals at the Fortune Theatre, Drury Lane, in the 1930s.

Her reaction to the operation and throughout her 'illness' was to talk about it briefly, optimistically and then switch to happier matters. She lost her brown, slightly greying hair and bravely wore a wig until the hair re-grew. For a few years she seemed healthy but suddenly she lost the use of her right arm. At this time she and I were both anxious and she was no longer able to distract herself with activities.

My father, always somewhat highly strung, seemed to cope adequately. At this time he learned the basics of cooking and willingly did most of the housework. He and my mother took many holidays but their plans for a retirement of walking and travelling were limited by her decreasing energy. He never complained.

My brother and I followed their lead, remaining calm; avoiding details that my father, particularly, did not wish to discuss; organizing and participating in family gatherings.

Mum attended the Royal Marsden regularly and we knew she was in good hands. She regained the use of her arm but there was another setback when her vital drugs induced a rare skin complaint. She was admitted to the New London Hospital in Whitechapel. Despite treatment, this problem never disappeared.

For the whole family the most traumatic event – one which still angers me unbearably – occurred when Mum developed pneumonia. Cancer had caused curvature of the spine so breathing was difficult. She was in pain and seriously deteriorating. We visited her in Mount Vernon Hospital. There were clear indications that she might die. Somehow, the doctors 'saved' her. I never discussed this with my dad but my husband and I, my brother and his wife all felt this to be the greatest cruelty. They should have let her go.

She transferred to the adjacent Macmillan Hospice. I was enormously impressed by the staff there but unutterably distressed as I listened to two adult sisters pleading with a doctor: 'You would have put down a dog when it was in half the pain our mum's enduring.' Indeed I had heard her constant moans.

Mum came home. Father had to turn her, lift her on to a commode and daily change dressings on the bleeding skin which was the manifestation of the rare disease. Mum had regressed almost to childhood. She had a teddy in bed and spoke to us in a light, remote voice. In 1987 she died peacefully at home. Father died of prostate cancer in 1991.

I remain convinced that the carer suffers hugely – their own life shattered, as much by sustained physical and psychological effort as by the ultimate loss of the loved one.

During the years of my mother's cancer I was a full-time secondary teacher with a husband and two children to care for. In addition, my love of theatre meant that I took many school trips to London and elsewhere and spent much time and energy co-ordinating large 'senior ' musicals. Mum was 90 minutes away. I visited often but in all our conversations we never discussed whether I was doing breast checks, to avoid the late detection she experienced. I was not. Inherited cancer was something neither of us had heard of.

Nevertheless, in the years after her death I worried about myself. I began to read articles on the subject in magazines – something I had assiduously avoided before. In 1992, I was eligible for the newly introduced NHS mammogram service. I badgered my doctor. Superstitiously I believed that anyone who is sensible enough to go for regular checks would be rewarded by avoiding the illness.

In September 1992, after my mammogram, I was stunned to receive a letter asking me to go for a re-test at the Churchill Hospital, Oxford. I told colleagues at school – my afternoon's absence was not cloaked in secrecy. They reassured me that a fault in the original X-ray was most common. But a colleague of the same age had just had a mastectomy and I was deeply worried. Still, my life had been punctuated by times of concealed panic for what had resolved itself as a harmless situation. This would surely be the same?

I drove 45 minutes to the hospital alone. If something is likely to be emotionally difficult I prefer to cope on my own. I have never been one to have a friend beside me on every occasion. I do not like to create a drama from a situation (except when I am in the acting studios!). An X-ray was followed by a biopsy – I did not even know what the word meant. It was unexpectedly painful, but I distracted myself by chatting to the young supervising doctor who, it transpired, had attended the same school as my children. The female consultant then accompanied me to her comfortable room. She showed me the X-ray, commented on how minute was the cluster of cells and then told me quietly that they were malignant.

I cannot fault my experience that day. She rapidly explained that surgery was necessary but that it would scarcely alter the shape of my breast. Mastectomy was not mentioned. I could have the operation in Oxford or in my home town with the experienced surgeon she recommended. I realized that I did not want to disrupt my working life – I wanted to have it done at half-term. She, a mother herself, would be away then. In any case I have warm feelings for my own hospital in which many friends work and where I had stayed only for the births of my two children.

At school I explained the situation to friends and made light of it. Indeed part of me felt very lucky – I had always thought there was a high chance I would have cancer someday. I had, and it had been detected early. My mind informed my emotions, telling me,'You can do nothing useful except to follow, intelligently and calmly, the prescribed course of action.'

Good – the cancer was non-invasive; but to be honest this made little sense since if it were malignant then it was surely dangerous? However, there was to be a short course of radiation as a precaution. Neither chemotherapy nor tamoxifen was deemed necessary. I could even laugh at the linguistic stupidity of 'lumpectomy' – a lumpen, Anglo-Saxon word lacking the style of the usual Greek medical terms.

I concentrated on believing that I had been let off lightly and got on with my work. I was further reassured when, on the day of the operation, it was necessary, because the lump was so small, to X-ray the breast and put a marker pin in place so that the surgeon knew where to cut. I joked with him about this – one of my ways of coping. However, the memory of Mum's cancer made me insist, contrary to the surgeon's plan, that a lymph sample was taken. It was clear, but the arm was awkward and nerve-ends dead for many months after.

Three days later I left hospital, spent the remainder of half-term recuperating and returned to school. My radiotherapy began some weeks later. Four minutes' exposure three times a week. I was very fortunate that a colleague offered to drive me. The 90-minute return journey after school plus effects of radiotherapy was more tiring than I realized – and the wasted appearance of some of the older patients was terribly depressing. Throughout this time family and friends helped me. My husband was more concerned than he showed but he remained calm and reassuring and, importantly, relieved me of all the household chores. The children, both away – one at university, the other working – kept in touch, came home, did not overdramatize it.

As the generations do now, we talked far more openly than I had with my mother. I always talked about it briefly and without, I hope, too much emotion. I did not want to embarrass or distress people; rather, I wanted cancer and its treatment to be accepted more easily into conversation. I wanted people to know that it could happen, that women could attend the mammogram centres, be treated and then be well. After all, I was now going to be monitored by an annual 'manual'(!) and X-ray plus ultrasound.

Then another colleague had a mastectomy – that made three of us. We each had different treatment, drugs prescribed or not prescribed, HRT forbidden or, in my case, the decision left to the patient. Such variation is confusing, even worrying. I coped by questioning specialists at the time, by exchanging information with others and, above all, continuing life on the basis that it will continue.

Having said that, I wasn't unaffected – my philosophy changed. I continued to work for five years after the operation, as I wanted to prove that cancer does not mean the sudden end of your usual life. But I was increasingly aware that I wanted more time to do as I wished. I valued family and friends more deeply and wanted to spend relaxed time with them. More selfishly, I wanted to do something different with my life.

I am proud of certain things I had already achieved: my family, my children's curiosity for life, the things they have achieved; proud that I was winched down Gaping Ghyll, crawled to Mud Hall, did the Lyke Wake Walk overnight; and even more that I have co-directed musicals and plays. But at 55 I was not sure what I wanted apart from a change and to travel.

Then an inheritance provided the answer. I took early retirement and was able to buy a derelict farmhouse in France, a country in which we have spent many holidays. My French was sufficient to cope with the basics of purchase and renovation. I was so pleased with myself – my husband had dealt with such things in the past.

The routine of life in south-west France and the physical nature of renovation mean that my focus is entirely different. It is challenging and it is fun. But I do talk of my cancer if the occasion arises. It keeps it in perspective, avoids melodrama, it helps reduce suppressed fears. For I have fears. One is that I may have a propensity to cancer so it may develop again; the other is what best should be done if, by chance, my daughter inherited the crucial genes. Neither of us is in favour of taking sudden, pre-emptive action.

There are so many women still working, or still relaxing, years after their operations. Last summer I was on a hot hillside bent between rows of vines, trying to harvest grapes as efficiently as my younger, newly acquired friend. As she straightened and wiped grape juice across her face she said, 'Who'd have thought I'd be here, doing this, ten years after my breast operation!' They are everywhere – women who faced the dread words: 'It is malignant!' The more you meet, the more confident you feel.

If you should hear those words for the first time, accept that good treatment is available and plan for the future. We are not all cut out to make amazing changes in our life but we will find a happier, more comfortable way to live. I do not mind if what I do is not 'mainstream' or if people do not fully understand why I am doing it. I shall continue to enjoy and absorb the French language and the quirks of French life. I shall continue to give more time to my husband and children – when they want me to! I'm just glad I'm here to say it.

Pamela's tips for surviving treatment

- Believe that you are receiving the best possible treatment, then it will work.
- Continue life as normally as possible so that you retain a balanced perspective.

Dedicated to my mother, Doris Taff

JUDY RICH

'You don't get to choose how you are going to die. Or when. You can only decide how you are going to live. Now.'
Joan Baez

Judy Rich, 56, is the Founder and Chairman of Long Tall Sally, established in 1976. She was born in Philadelphia, Pennsylvania, USA, and lives in London with her husband Richard and son William, 15.

Judy was diagnosed with breast cancer in 1988, aged 44, following a routine Well Woman screening. She had a lumpectomy, followed by six weeks of radiotherapy and four months of chemotherapy at the Princess Grace Hospital and the Cromwell Hospital, London.

Judy's Story

Nothing prepares you for the shock of discovering you have breast cancer. Even with a history in the family, you somehow feel it won't get you as you sail through the glorious days of your twenties and thirties feeling immortal. My mother died of breast cancer, so I was aware of the hereditary factor. This was underlined for me when I married my English husband in the United States, where you needed a blood test and routine medical examination before you got a marriage licence. The fatherly doctor who checked me over and took my family history cautioned me to have regular breast checks. Here I was in an ecstatic state of happiness at my upcoming wedding – life was beautiful, full of promise – I didn't want to think about breast cancer. That was 1983 . . . I was 39.

My life has been eventful since I moved to London in 1974. At nearly six feet tall, I shopped in London's exciting boutiques and markets but despaired of finding fashionable clothes that fit me. Shopping for clothes had always been a nightmare for me and I dreamed of a store where everything would be long enough, where there would be plenty of choice and where being tall would be an asset, not a burden. I shared my vision with a friend of mine, a businessman, and he offered to back me – lending me the money and giving me sound business advice. The first Long Tall Sally opened in London in 1976 and I have never looked back. It seemed thousands of women in Britain shared my predicament, and today, Long Tall Sally is the market leader of clothes for tall women, with 25 stores, a mail order service and 200,000 tall women on our mailing list.

Meeting and marrying my husband and having a beautiful baby boy at 40 was the culmination of everything I had ever hoped for. There I was, fulfilling every dream, the business was successful and I was very busy. I was 43 years old with a three-year-old son when the lump in my breast was discovered. Fortunately, I'd taken the advice of the wise US doctor and started having regular mammograms at a Well Woman clinic in London. I'd almost cancelled my last appointment – life was so full, I had so much to do – but I managed to squeeze it into my busy schedule. 'Benign fibroid adenoma,' said the radiologist; 'come back in six months.' I breathed a sigh of relief . . . but only for a few moments. 'I have a history of breast cancer in the family,' I said. 'I think I should see a specialist.' My GP agreed, referred me immediately, and within five days I was in the Princess Grace Hospital having a malignant lump removed.

I checked into the hospital armed with a pile of books from the alternative bookstore. I wanted to know what was being written, researched, experienced and talked about with regard to breast cancer. I knew I was getting excellent and efficient medical care, but I wanted to know what else was being written about breast cancer. I read about diet, nutrition, vitamins, relaxation, and many alternative ideas for complementary treatment of breast cancer. What felt right to me, I put into my recovery programme. I knew I was a Type A personality – prone to always being on the go, so a course in relaxation proved invaluable. Watching my diet seemed sensible and a visit to the Bristol Cancer Help Centre set me on a course of healthy eating and vitamins to combat what my body was losing through radiation and chemotherapy. Making choices and finding positive things I could do to help myself made me feel better and more in

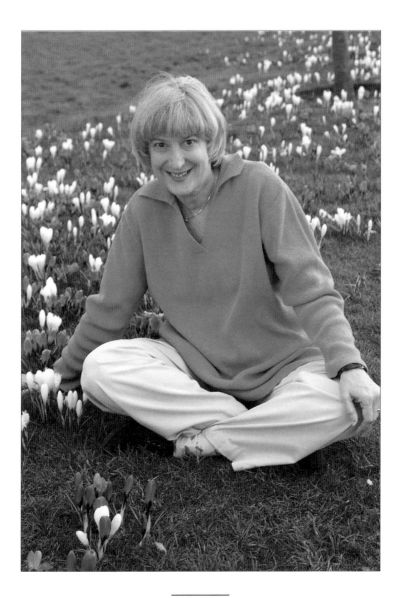

Judy Rich

charge of my body. It seemed to balance out in a gentle way all the invasive and drastic measures that were being taken to kill the cancer cells. I was doing things for me – not just waiting for things to be done to me.

One of the most startling statistics I came across in my reading was that the mortality rate for breast cancer had remained virtually unchanged since my mother had died of the disease over 25 years earlier. While modern medicine improved life expectancy, 15,000 women a year were dying of breast cancer in the UK alone. I was shocked and, like many women affected by the disease either directly or indirectly, I felt the need to act!

I was in the middle of chemotherapy when a friend told me about a new charity being created to build a centre focusing exclusively on breast cancer research with the hope of finding a cure. When I heard about this charity – Breakthrough Breast Cancer – I knew this was where I wanted to put my energies and the resources of my company, Long Tall Sally. After all, we were a company run by women, for women and with 200,000 women on our mailing list; there was plenty of scope for raising awareness and funds to fight breast cancer.

Breakthrough became our company charity and we spread the word through our mail order catalogues and in all our stores. All of us at Long Tall Sally have had a lot of fun raising money. Our staff have held auctions, raffles and car boot sales galore, had bowling parties, fashion shows and disco evenings. We've held sponsored walks and sponsored pub crawls, jumped out of airplanes and, most recently, Long Tall Sally sponsored and joined in the Breakthrough Women's Challenge – a unique opportunity for women to discover the thrill of outdoor adventure while raising money for breast cancer. Our slogan for this event neatly sums up my current inspirational motto: 'Go on . . . life's too short . . . not to!'

Being involved with Breakthrough has given my life a purpose and a direction that has been rewarding, exciting and challenging. It puts me in touch with women from all walks of life who share my experience of breast cancer, either directly or indirectly, and who are taking a proactive stand to make a difference in the world. I love the sense of sisterhood and teamwork that develops around the breast cancer campaign. I've cycled 30 miles, held many a Breakthrough breakfast, organized friends for Breakthrough walks and, while none of these activities raises 'big bucks', they go a long way in bringing women together to celebrate life and just 'be'.

My advice to anyone facing the terrifying experience of breast cancer is: get on with your life as much as possible. I knew that after chemotherapy sessions (on Wednesdays), Thursday would be a lost day with sickness and feeling wasted, but by Friday I'd be back in the real world . . . if a little shattered and very fragile. We would always plan to go away that weekend – to friends, to the country. It was hard to get motivated but it beat lying in bed feeling sorry for myself. My husband, close friends and family were terrific. While I knew they were worried and concerned, they didn't let me see too much of that and encouraged me to just get on with things.

I'm truly proud of my life so far. Thanks to Long Tall Sally, I've been able to fulfil a dream of having fantastic clothes to fit . . . as well as providing that opportunity for thousands of tall women in Britain. And using this audience and the resources of the company, I've been able to raise awareness of breast cancer as well as raise thousands of pounds towards the fight against breast cancer.

Lately I've been asked to speak about my personal experiences and Breakthrough so I have had to face another life challenge – public speaking. While I always enjoyed being behind the scenes, now I was being asked to 'speak up'. It was daunting – but it was an opportunity to grow that I seized despite the butterflies in my stomach. And if it helps others to come to terms with breast cancer or inspires people to take up the crusade to fight it – then I'll continue to speak out.

There's still a lot I want to do and life still feels very precious. It is twelve years since I had my breast cancer experience and I know I am one of the lucky ones. I struggle with remaining in the present and valuing every minute and not letting anticipation or worry about the future run my life. Every day is precious and who knows what the future will be. I'd like to take on a physical challenge, climb a mountain or go on a long trek. I'd like to mentor other women who are starting up in business. I'd like to have more time for watercolours, reading, my family and friends. I'm 56 years young! My mother never reached this age and yet she must have felt just like me. Breast cancer strikes too many women in the prime of life. More than anything else, I'd like to help find that cure.

Judy's tip for surviving treatment

Look for things that inspire or excite you to help you through the long treatment process.

Judy's book recommendations

Love, Medicine and Miracles by Bernie Siegel

Prescriptions for Living by Bernie Siegel

Dedicated to my youngest sister, Suzie Rich, who is also facing the challenge of breast cancer in her life

MYRA POWELL

Think young like your children and move with the younger generation.

Myra Powell, 68, lives in Castleton, Derbyshire, with her husband Les. She has a son, Russell, 42, two daughters, Lesley-Ann, 39, and Jenny, 32, and three grandchildren, Jonathan, Lana and Sam.

Myra was diagnosed with breast cancer in 1992, aged 59. She had an invasive ductal carcinoma with no lymph nodes involved for which she received a mastectomy at the Royal Hospital in Calow, Chesterfield, Derbyshire. Myra took tamoxifen for five years.

Myra's Story

It takes something like breast cancer to make you realize how precious your life is. In the eighties I was working for a shipping company. All the female staff were sent to a Well Woman clinic run by BUPA. This included a mammogram. I must have been about 48 years old then. They discovered a shadow in my left breast and I was then sent to the Royal Marsden Hospital for further consultation and had check-ups for about two years. Then as no lump had appeared during this period I was given the all-clear.

Life went on. Then my husband and I decided to retire and we moved from the South to Derbyshire, to enjoy the lovely countryside and to live a slower pace of life. We left behind most of the family, including my son Russell, my daughter Lesley-Ann and my grandson, Jonathan. We moved to a lovely village called Castleton, in an area quite near to my younger daughter, Jenny. I found myself a part-time job working in a gift shop among very friendly people.

In 1992, I was due for a routine mammogram, the first since the one at BUPA, and attended the usual screening, feeling very confident as I could not feel or see any lump – but at the back of my mind I still remembered the shadow in my left breast. I can remember saying to my husband, 'I won't be surprised if they call me back as the shadow could still possibly be there, but don't worry, I have no lump after all these years.'

Well, shortly after the screening I received a letter, asking me to attend the Royal Hospital in Chesterfield to see the cancer consultant. The results showed the shadow was still there and needed further investigation. The consultant suggested I come back after three months for a second screening, to see if there were any changes in the shape of the shadow.

I continued working and enjoying my job among my friends – it took my mind off the problem and I was still confident all was well because there was no lump. The person who needed reassuring was my husband (he is a born worrier). After three months I had another screening and this did show a change in the shape of the shadow. I was shown the X-ray and could see the difference. It was then that I started to become slightly concerned. It was suggested that I have a biopsy within the next few days, which entailed a general anaesthetic and an overnight stay in hospital. This was quite painless and all I had was a couple of stitches.

I returned to my job – still not really worried. Working probably helped to keep my mind occupied. If my husband and children were concerned at this stage they certainly never showed it. The thought that there was no actual lump was some consolation to me. After one week I went back to see my consultant to see the results of my biopsy. I was told the tissue they had removed had started to go malignant. My husband, who was waiting in the reception room, was called in to join us to discuss the next procedure.

My husband was in a state of shock and very emotional – but a sudden feeling of calmness came over me. Maybe this happens when you are a mother and your instincts are to protect the ones you love – and I knew that I had to be strong for my family.

My consultant was a very caring and wonderful man and I felt I could put my trust in him. We spoke quite frankly to each other. He gave me two options: either to have all the malignant tissue removed and have an intensive course of radiotherapy, or to have a mastectomy. He suggested that we go home and discuss this but without doubt, I made up my mind then and there that I was going to have a mastectomy. After all, this was my body. My family was complete and as I had gone through menopause (luckily with no problems) my breast was just a lump of muscle which would serve no further purpose – I just wanted to enjoy the rest of my life.

We went home to speak to the children and tell them of my decision. We asked them all to help me by being very positive and to deal with each stage of my treatment as it happened. My daughter Jenny was the only family member who lived close by. Russell and Lesley-Ann lived in the South so we spoke on the telephone – but they were all very supportive. Within the next few days I was in surgery for a mastectomy.

The most amusing thing about all this was that my consultant (bless him) was so aware of my husband's distress and concern for me that when I came round in the recovery room, he came to tell me that everything had gone well and that he was going to find my husband immediately, to tell him the same thing. To this very day, when I attend my yearly check-up, he still asks my husband if he is OK!

I've had wonderful aftercare. I've had three prostheses – they do tend to split after two years. All I do is phone the clinic, see the nurse and I am supplied with a new one. My lifestyle has not altered a bit. I was back to work after three months and I went on holiday to Cyprus after two months. Nobody could tell I had had a mastectomy. My friends and family have been no different in their attitude towards me. I am treated normally. In fact, at times I think they tend to forget I have had cancer! New people I meet don't know unless the topic arises in conversation and I always mention that I had breast cancer because I do not believe in holding back. Talking helps you heal and forget. When I was a teenager my parents tended not to mention the 'Big C' just as they never mentioned TB.

My priorities in life now are to eat healthily, have lots of vegetables and exercise. Think young like your children and move with the younger generation. Also, I am learning to swim at the age of 68 and I am determined to master this!

I am very proud of my husband Les and my children and the rest

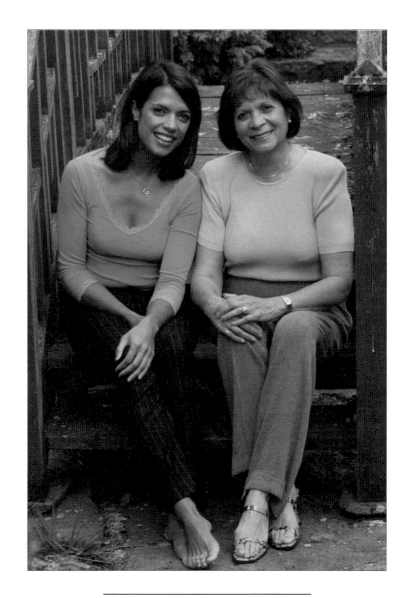

Myra Powell with daughter Jenny

of the family. They acted exactly as I asked them to, at the beginning of my illness and throughout, with lots of encouragement and care, just being themselves. I now have three grandchildren whom I adore and thank God that I am here to enjoy them all. I never look at myself and feel horrible about my body – I am thankful just to wake up every morning and think I could easily have not been here. Minor aches and pains do not worry me, or whether the sun is shining outside. My husband calls me 'my one-titty girl' and we laugh about that.

Myra's tips for surviving treatment

- Be positive and talk about it to your friends if it helps you to relax.
- Deal with each stage at a time and don't worry about the unknown.

Dedicated to Rita, my sister-in-law, who has been suffering from breast cancer for the last four years. She does not complain although she is in constant pain. I believe her strong faith in her religion sees her through.

EILEEN ATKINS

I can fasten on a beautiful day, as a bee fixes itself on a sunflower. It feeds me, rests me, satisfies me, as nothing else does . . . This has a holiness. This will go on after I am dead.

THE DIARY OF VIRGINIA WOOLF, *1932*

Eileen Atkins, 66, is an award-winning stage actress and writer for film and television, including *Upstairs, Downstairs* and *The House of Eliott*. She lives in London with her husband, producer Bill Shepherd.

Eileen was diagnosed with breast cancer in 1995, aged 61, at the Sloane Kettering Hospital in New York. She had a lumpectomy at the same hospital, followed by six months of chemotherapy and radiotherapy at the Royal Marsden Hospital, London.

Eileen's Story

In 1995, I was playing on Broadway in Cocteau's *Les Parents terribles* (called *Indiscretions* in America, a French title being thought not good for business) when I discovered I had breast cancer.

I was undressing for bed and, as I took off my bra, I thought, 'How odd, my breast feels as it used to before a period.' I put my hand to my right breast and found a lump. It was after 2 a.m. so there was no one I could call, nothing I could do, until the morning. I had two shows to do the next day so I had to get to sleep.

The minute I arrived at the theatre for the matinée, I rushed to the stage management office and said, 'I have a lump in my breast. Call our producer, he knows everyone, and tell him to get me an appointment with one of the best breast cancer specialists, first thing Monday morning.' They calmly said they'd call him, and then said a fax had just come through for me. The first two lines of the fax read: 'Caroline is getting married and Pat found Hayley's knickers in John's bed – disgusting I call it!'

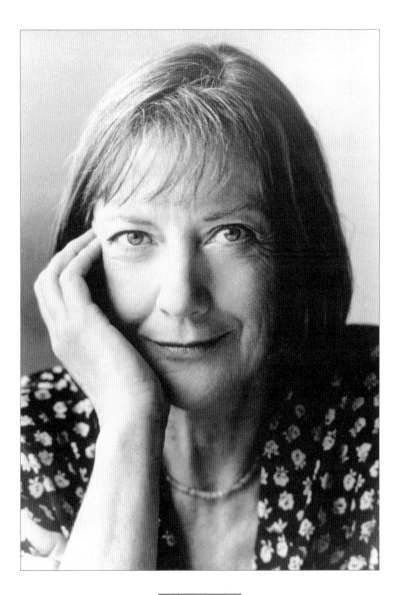

Eileen Atkins

'What the hell is this?' I shrieked. That was when I realized I was tense. It was a summary of what had been happening in *The Archers* that Judi Dench sometimes sends me, with her own comments on life in Ambridge. Her timing has always been perfect.

I had an appointment at 10 a.m. on Monday at Sloane Kettering Hospital with an oncologist with the delightful name of Chips Cody. I went to the hospital alone. I find it better to go alone. You don't have to put on a performance for anyone or worry about them. Better to have an engrossing book to read.

Almost immediately he touched the lump, Cody told me he was sure that it was cancer. To my surprise, my first thoughts and words were: 'Well, at least that means I won't have to do the play any more.' I had been playing *Indiscretions* for five months, but I'd done it back to back – that is, rehearsing in the day while still playing in the evenings – with another play of my own with Vanessa Redgrave; so I had been performing eight times a week for over a year, and had also written the film script of *Mrs Dalloway* during the day. I was very tired and part of me was longing to get back to England and my husband.

At the end of all the tests, the lump was confirmed as cancerous. Cody recommended an immediate lumpectomy and said he would take some lymph glands as well, in case the cancer had reached them, but he was 99 per cent sure it hadn't. It would mean only radiotherapy after the operation. I had planned to fly back to London but the producer persuaded me to stay and have the surgery and radiotherapy in New York. Afterwards I could go back into the show. I was under contract for nine months so I felt duty-bound to try.

My husband flew out to New York and I had the operation a week later. The day before the surgery, my blood pressure shot up. 'Try and calm down,' said the very camp young man from the South who was taking it. 'I can't calm down,' I said, rather tetchy. 'I'm having an operation tomorrow, and I'm terrified.' 'Miss Atkins,' came the droll voice, 'you're having the teensy-weensiest operation we do in this hospital.' That calmed me down.

The operation was fine. The hospital stay itself was a nightmare. Four televisions on at full blast, all on different stations, immediately outside my room, and mainly for the entertainment of the staff.

The next day, a counsellor breezed into my room and said, 'You must be very angry.' 'What? Oh, you mean they've told you I went crazy last night with all the televisions going at full blast,' I said. 'No. You're angry that you've got cancer.' 'Why would I be angry?' 'Because you're thinking, "Why me?"' 'I've spent most of my life thinking, "Why not me?" so why on earth shouldn't it be me now?'

Five days later I went back to the hospital to have the drain removed and to get the results of my biopsy. It was a blow. They had found cancer in my lymph glands. Now, six months of chemotherapy and then radiotherapy lay ahead of me. It was my lowest point – but at least now I could go home.

The next morning Mike Nichols called me. 'You should speak to Susan Sontag,' he said. The last person in the world I wanted to speak to was Susan Sontag, a brilliant, formidable intellectual, who I'd briefly met once. She turned up at 9.30 a.m., chain-smoking as she talked and told me she'd been diagnosed with breast cancer 25 years before: both breasts, a double mastectomy, cancer found in all lymph glands and she'd been given three to six months to live – no point in chemotherapy.

So she rang everyone she knew and found an oncologist in Paris who said he would take her on. She had chemotherapy continually for two years, lost her hair and grew it back, three times, recovered and wrote a book: *Illness as Metaphor*.

Now, she was involved in several projects, including directing a play in Sarajevo, flying in and out in the worst bombing – in fact, she was flying back that afternoon. She hadn't had cosmetic surgery on her breasts, although she admitted she didn't like looking at the scars much.

'You won't believe me,' she said as she breezed off, 'but you'll feel slightly sad the day your chemotherapy ends.'

Until that moment I'd never understood why people needed role models, but I thought, 'My God, if she can go through all that and not only pull through, but be so amazingly active 25 years later – she was in her mid-sixties – then I can jolly well pull through.'

I came home and started my treatment at the Royal Marsden under the utterly charming, calming Dr Ian Smith. I knew absolutely nothing about chemotherapy except that it made you very sick and you lost your hair.

'Well,' said Smith, 'you might not feel sick and you might not lose your hair – some women don't.' And I didn't lose my hair and I only felt nauseous a couple of times.

My chemotherapy nurse, Dawn Davis, was a lovely, bright (indeed brilliant) young woman who I gossiped and laughed with all the way through the treatment. The atmosphere in the chemotherapy room was comforting and never gloomy. A woman once asked us to be quiet as she was trying to think beautiful thoughts. I whispered rather loudly that the thought of Sting, who we were discussing, was a beautiful enough thought. Silly – but the woman was pretentious.

I met many interesting people in the chemotherapy room. There was a young woman of 22 who did lose all her hair. She dressed from top to toe in leather and confessed to me that she had been a rather shy person, somewhat bullied on the council estate where she lived – but when she lost her hair, people took it for granted she was a skinhead, and were nervous of her, so she decided to dress the part, and said that she now had a lot more confidence.

I met a man who was a journalist, who wore a contraption round his waist that continuously gave him chemotherapy, but he had to pop in from time to time to get topped up – he was off to work in Afghanistan that evening.

I was contracted, before I was ill, to play in *John Gabriel Borkman* at the National Theatre. I had just enough time to complete my treatment before starting rehearsals. But anyway, as I was lucky and felt well most of the time, I got bored doing nothing and did some radio, read some novels for cassettes, and adapted another book for a film script. I lived quietly, avoided gloomy people and was through with the radiotherapy just in time. And Susan Sontag was right, I was slightly sad when it all stopped. I missed seeing Dawn every few weeks, I would miss seeing Ian Smith, I missed the other patients, their stories, the camaraderie.

Has the experience changed my life? I try to live more in the moment. I get more pleasure from simple things. I think I'm more philosophical, but my husband and friends probably wouldn't agree, although Maggie Smith did ring another friend of mine, Zoë Caldwell, and said, 'What's happened to Eileen? She's euphoric, and she used to be such a moaner!' 'That's how they get when they've had cancer,' came Zoë's answer!

Eileen's tips for surviving treatment

- Trust your oncologist. Whatever percentage chance he says you have of overcoming your cancer, decide to be in that percentage.

Eileen's book recommendation

- *The Diary of Virginia Woolf*

Dedicated to Susan Sontag

LOLLY SUSI

The only reason you're special is because your friends and family say you are. Who says it when you are on your own?

MARCIE IN GONE TO LA, LOLLY SUSI

Lolly Susi, 50, is an actress, director, teacher and writer from the US. Her first play, *Gone to LA,* has been produced by the Hampstead Theatre in London and her second, *The Perfect Truth*, is to be produced in the West End. Lolly most recently appeared in Tennessee Williams's *Orpheus Descending* with Helen Mirren at the Donmar Warehouse.

Lolly was diagnosed with breast cancer in 1995, aged 45, at the Middlesex Hospital, London. She had a Stage III tumour with ten lymph nodes involved. Following a lumpectomy and axillary clearance, she entered a trial for high-dose chemotherapy with stem-cell replacement. Six weeks of radiotherapy followed. She lives in London.

Lolly's Story

What You Always Wanted to Know about Cancer but Had Too Much Taste to Ask

I was diagnosed with breast cancer in September 1995. By the time I discovered my lump, the cancer had spread to my lymph glands. After surgery to remove the tumour and the ten affected glands, I went into a clinical trial, which offered high-dose chemotherapy with stem-cell self-transplantation, followed by six weeks of radiotherapy. From my diagnosis to the end of treatment was an intense eight months, to which was added approximately a year of post-treatment recovery. Since then, I have been stronger, busier, happier and perhaps healthier than I remember being for a long time. Through hard experience I learned that breast cancer is not necessarily a killer. It is, however, a gargantuan, rapacious, neck-throttling wake-up call. It is

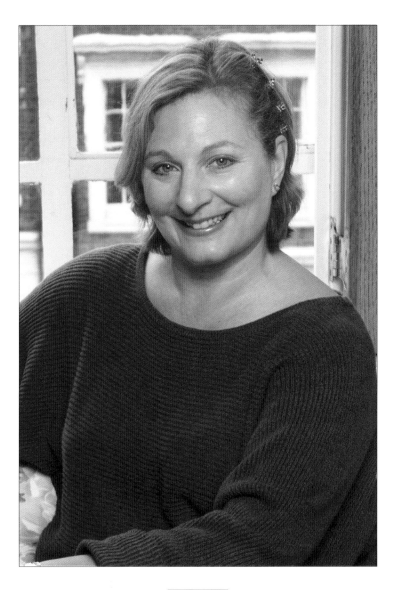

Lolly Susi

an intensive course in survival, a learning experience, a life lesson – and a gigantic pain in the backside.

Most of us live steady, predictable lives, punctuated by insignificant dramas: late buses or bad traffic or grey weather. If you are unfortunate enough to hear the words 'You have breast cancer', those luxurious minor inconveniences are left far behind and you instantly, urgently, need a whole new set of coping skills. I certainly was ill-prepared for what I faced, and I imagine this may be the case for many others. But now, having been through it all, from diagnosis to post-treatment follow-up visits, I am experienced. I am a 'veteran', a 'professional'. I feel as if I have earned a Ph.D. in Breast Cancer.

I think we may get the deepest benefit from cancer, as indeed from most cathartic life events, if we incessantly talk or write about it. It is perhaps imperative that we exhaust friends and family with stories of ill treatment at the hands of the medical professionals and share tirelessly the litany of aches and pains that accompany treatment (I like to think of this as an 'organ recital'). But, most importantly, I feel it is our obligation to bestow our hard-won wisdom upon others who, like us, have been thrust unarmed into an alien land. The cancer charities do a marvellous job of offering support and information, but it is up to us, the survivors, to share the day-to-day nitty-gritty lessons we have learned along the way.

So, for those of you who have already entered the wacky world of cancer, or for you who are trying to support someone who has, or perhaps even for those of you who are considering taking the plunge and getting cancer yourself, here are my 'Top Twenty Cancer Tips', or 'Things You Didn't Know You Needed to Know to Get Back to Your Life and Put This Nightmare Behind You':

1. If you have a morning appointment with a National Health consultant, do not make lunch plans.
2. If you have an appointment at a National Health clinic, don't make any plans – for a long, long time. Take a big book. Take a snack. Take water, a sleeping bag and photos of your loved ones.
3. If chemotherapy doesn't make you live longer, rest assured that, at the very least, it will seem longer.

4. Everyone who has never had cancer/chemotherapy knows one thing: 'It is important to be positive.'

5. Everyone who *has* had cancer/chemotherapy can tell you three things: One and two: 'It sucks to be sick all the time and have your hair fall out.' And three: 'Positive has nothing to do with it.'

6. Hair's a marvellous invention. Without it, your head gets cold and all your hats are too big.

7. Yes, when all of your hair falls out, all of your hair falls out.

8. Never pat a woman on the head – she may be wearing a wig. (If you knock off her wig, she may knock off something of yours.)

9. If you're wearing a wig and your head itches, use one hand to anchor and the other to scratch, otherwise the whole mess will move around all over the place and you'll resemble an alien only here on earth to collect soil samples.

10. If you're nauseous, all coloured foods are strictly forbidden. Stick to beige. No substitutions.

11. Everybody's cancer is different. Aunty Mary will not necessarily die just because your neighbour did (no matter how much you dislike Aunty Mary and desperately want to be an heiress).

12. Everyone who visits hospital has had a 'nightmare journey' to get there. If you are the visitor, please keep this information to yourself. It's possible that the real nightmare is not the 'journey', but the 'already being there'.

13. Hospital visitors should remember that parking near hospitals can be expensive and difficult to find. Cancer patients either (a) already know this, or (b) don't care, so please think of something else to share with them during your hopefully short visit.

14. Long hospital visits should be for close family and friends only. (Think of the savings on parking.)

15. One's partiality to grapes is not exponentially increased by the seriousness of one's illness.

16. Cancer is only 'in remission' if it belongs to someone else. If it is your cancer, consider it 'cured'.

17. Beet juice is a highly overrated beverage and should be banned by the government for tasting like dirt.

18. You probably know that life isn't a dress rehearsal. But did you

know that it has a limited run and can be closed without a two-week notice?

19. Life is too short to not do what you want to do.
20. Life is too short to live without love or laughter. It's too short to be insecure, or unhappy, or judgemental, or scared. It's far, far too short to go without ice cream or chocolate.

I suppose I could offer more serious tips: (1) drink plenty of water after chemotherapy to flush the chemicals out of your bladder, or (2) if you vomit after chemo, always, always rinse with a strong mouthwash to prevent mouth ulcers. But I think I'll leave that sort of thing to the medical experts. I only hope my advice will prove helpful to those looking for answers to questions they haven't thought of yet. If it hasn't been helpful, then I hope that at the very least it has made you smile. I, for one, feel a lot better for sharing with you. Wisdom, after all, best satisfies the wise when thrust enthusiastically at anyone who will sit still long enough. As a matter of fact, I feel so good that, after I brush my hair, I think I'll treat myself to a wide array of brightly coloured foods. And a large, large bowl of chocolate ice cream.

Lolly's tips for surviving treatment

- ❀ I embraced as many alternative therapies as I could afford during my treatment.
- ❀ I took time to relax, eat well and give myself as many treats as possible, and tried to laugh a lot!

Lolly's book recommendation

- ❀ *Dr Susan Love's Breast Book*

Cancer is not a gift. Life is a gift. Cancer merely reminds us of that.

Dedicated to my brother, Peter Susi, who came to England to be with me for my high-dose chemo. His irrepressible sense of humour made a gruesome experience bearable.

LIZA GODDARD

The world is a stage, but the play is badly cast.

LADY WINDERMERE'S FAN, *OSCAR WILDE*

Liza Goddard, 50, is a well-known actor on stage and television and has starred in award-winning programmes such as *Take Three Girls*, *Woof!*, *Skippy* and *Bergerac*. She lives in Norfolk with her husband, producer and director David Cobham, and three dogs, Mina, Cassie and Chloe. She has a son, Thomas, 24, a daughter, Sophie, 18, and a grand-daughter, Adelaide, 8 months.

Liza was diagnosed with breast cancer in 1997, aged 47, at the Norfolk and Norwich Hospital. She had a DCIS (ductal carcinoma *in situ* – a non-invasive tumour) for which she had a lumpectomy, followed by 30 sessions of radiotherapy, at the same hospital. She currently takes tamoxifen.

Liza's Story

Life seems to be a series of problems that have to be sorted out. Obstacles need to be overcome. Nobody's life is easy. There are moments in your life when you think, 'I can't cope with this' – it's almost as if you have too many problems – but somehow these periods pass and you get an easier time. But there are always problems to be confronted and sorted – and that's what life is.

But the good parts in life far outweigh the bad. The only problem is that life goes so quickly. Here I am at 50 and I can't believe it. The last 25 years have gone in a flash. Appreciate what you have got now, each day – because life just whizzes past.

Cancer makes you appreciate what you have much more and, of course, it makes you realize that you are mortal, that there is a definite end to your life instead of it going on for ever. You never think about it normally.

My having cancer was hard on the family. It was very hard on David. He was away filming at the time and was very worried. He had dealt with cancer – a skin melanoma – himself. But everyone was helpful and supportive. In a way, it is easier for the person having the treatment for cancer, because you've got things to do, places to go, people to see. You get caught up in this world, this 'cancer world', and you're very active but the people at home just sit and worry. David always came on all my appointments with me – to the radiotherapy and to see the oncologists. But husbands are normally just considered an appendage and no one takes their feelings into consideration.

A friend, Jane, said the most helpful thing anyone could say to me about the treatment: 'Radiotherapy is a breeze.' I had that gleaming like a beacon in my mind. It helped me get through it, because it implies that the whole thing is a breeze, if you have the right attitude. It means you take control of your body. You monitor what you eat, take lots of vitamins and have reflexology and aromatherapy, if it makes you feel better and more positive. I had acupuncture and took vitamins because I thought that if I could make my immune system really strong I would recover more quickly from the effects of radiotherapy and indeed I did. I was working again at the theatre in a couple of weeks following treatment. I kept falling asleep at four o'clock in the afternoon and wanted to sleep in the middle of a scene but I kept going – you just keep going.

I do find mammograms painful, however. I'm totally phobic about them and I'm getting worse. Men have no idea about mammogram machines. They should stick their balls in them! Then they might have an idea how painful it is and design a better machine. A girlfriend of mine had a brilliant idea. She said what they ought to do is make a machine so that you lie on your front and there's a hole that you can drop your boobs through. The whole thing about squashing them is because you're standing up – if you are lying down your boobs would go forward so you're not trying to reverse gravity, as it were.

Now the treatment is over I am probably more spiritual. You realize things don't matter nearly so much. In my business you see people getting terribly upset about their costumes and their wigs, and it's good to get things right but, on the other hand, it doesn't really matter – it's only a play.

I do still get frightened on the first night, though. My first-night quote is 'It's better than an enema.' That's because everyone's frightened and it's catching and it gets worse and worse. You're standing on the side of the stage with your heart pumping through your body, longing for a heart attack or some major illness so you can be carried away in an ambulance. It's got to be something serious – you can't just faint. You stand there thinking this is a silly way of earning a living. What can I do instead? . . . coming up with nothing. It's pure fear running through your body. On first nights my legs shake, and I remember saying to someone about my diagnosis and treatment, 'It's not as bad as a first night.'

I want to make my life much more simple now. The children have left home and I don't want to work so much. I want to spend more time with David and travel more when he retires: 'To live life entirely for pleasure,' as Lady Bracknell in Oscar Wilde's *The Importance of Being Earnest* says. When the children were young and at school, it was all work, work, work to feed them and clothe them and educate them. Now we think we are going to sit back a bit, just take the odd job that's important – otherwise be home and walk the dogs.

My best achievement is bringing up the children – making sure they were educated. I'm very proud of them. I'm also proud of my career – *Woof!*, *Skippy* and *Take Three Girls*, the first ever drama series to be filmed in colour as well as the first series to star three girls in the lead roles. I've had a varied career – comedy to light drama. I've been lucky. My big ambition was to play Lady Bracknell – now I've done it so maybe I'd like to play all of Oscar Wilde's plays. It's a precarious profession but I've always done different things.

In this career you have to wait and see what comes along. I take whatever's offered – I've played a lot of the great roles. I have a saying: 'Yesterday's history, tomorrow's a mystery, live for today!'

Meanwhile, my ambition now is to keep bees. I'm reading up on them and when we're settled I'm going to keep them. My role model is my aunt in West Sussex who keeps bees. The bees love her and

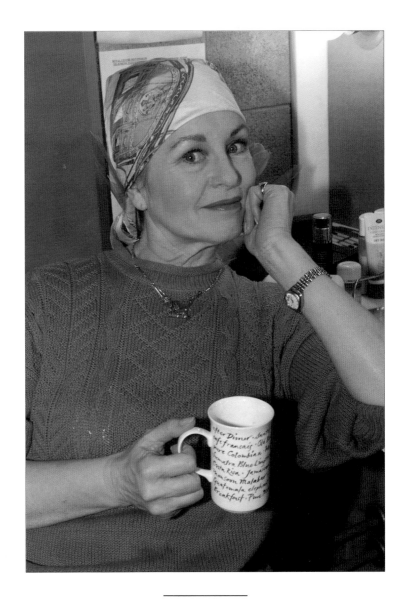

Liza Goddard

come up to her and kiss her. I think you need to be calm to keep bees and I want to be like that.

Liza's tips for surviving treatment

- You must think positive.
- You must take charge of your body.
- Sleep. Some days I would be very negative and I'd go to bed for an hour. I'd feel depressed and down and I'd hide under the duvet with Mina, my dog. Then I'd get up and feel fine. It's a very good thing to have a sleep.

Liza's book recommendation

- *You Can Heal Your Life* by Louise Hay

We are all in the gutter but some of us are looking up at the stars.
LORD DARLINGTON IN LADY WINDERMERE'S FAN, OSCAR WILDE

Dedicated to David, Thom, Sophie and Adelaide

LINDA McDONALD

Life is no 'brief candle' to me. It is a sort of splendid torch which I have got hold of for a moment, and I want to make it burn as brightly as possible before handing it on to future generations.

'ART AND PUBLIC MONEY', GEORGE BERNARD SHAW

Linda McDonald, 53, works for StartHere, an innovative new information technology charity. She is also launching a new charity called Investors in Children. She has a daughter, Jo, 26, a son Andrew, 22, and a granddaughter, Dhiya, 3. She lives in Hampton, Middlesex.

Linda was diagnosed with breast cancer in 1994, aged 47, at the Royal Marsden Hospital, London. She had an invasive ductal carcinoma and underwent four months of chemotherapy, followed by a lumpectomy and six weeks of radiotherapy. She completed five years of taking tamoxifen in April 2000.

Linda's Story

For Margaret

Cancer – the word you hope you will never hear about yourself. You hear of other people who have it but it is something you never imagine can happen to you. I had a good friend with me, Annie, when they told me I had a tumour in my left breast. Was there something symbolic about it being near my heart, I thought to myself? Annie grabbed my hand and tears were in her eyes. I felt nothing. I became the 'star' in my own film, watching myself act out a role I hadn't learned. I waited for the script from these fine directors of my cancer, the heroes in white coats and pink frocks. They were going to be co-stars in my film, telling me what to do.

I became a little child again, realizing that the grown-ups knew more about my coming life than I could ever imagine.

I had choices. I chose to have a Hickman line, connected to an infusion box with batteries, that would continually pump the cancer-killers around my body for four months. I imagined great big Rottweilers living in that box and at night they would come out and eat the cancer out of my body. I would go into the Marsden, my own special film set, every three weeks for a mega-hit chemo-cocktail. I decided I would be one of their snowy bike riders and wear the ice-helmet to help prevent hair loss – I had just met a special man who was a fanatical motorbike rider so it seemed appropriate to match his hair-raising antics with my own hair-saving ones! My very short hair stayed mostly on my head and it made me feel so good.

I don't want to tell you about the hard times because every cancer person has them and they are different for everyone. A Walkman in hospital was a boon and writing a diary gave me a sense of achievement. I got through treatment by learning how to visualize and by muttering my mantras. I used positive thinking and I prayed to my God to walk beside me and beside those who loved me.

My friend Louise taught me to visualize and I was always in the Rocky Mountains, where I used to live. I walked through a valley of flowers with the forests and the mountains in the distance. My father – who died a few years before – came out of the forest towards me. He held out his arms to me and hugged me and I felt warm. He told me I was going to be fine and that he loved me, and then he turned round and disappeared into the forest.

When I was having radiotherapy and I was 'pinned down like a butterfly', I visualized Blackfoot Indian women and children (whom I had met) weaving me a fine cloak of feathers, and every time I went to radiotherapy the cloak got bigger until the last session, when they lined it with fur and closed it around me.

I walked around the house muttering, 'I am not going to be sick, I am never going to be sick. Sick? What me? No never!' They must have worked with the anti-sickness drug because I was only sick once and I am sure that is because I ate too many bananas! My favourite one for walking around Tesco was 'I am really well, I will always be well, wellness is with me, I am a well bunny.' People must have thought I had escaped from somewhere!

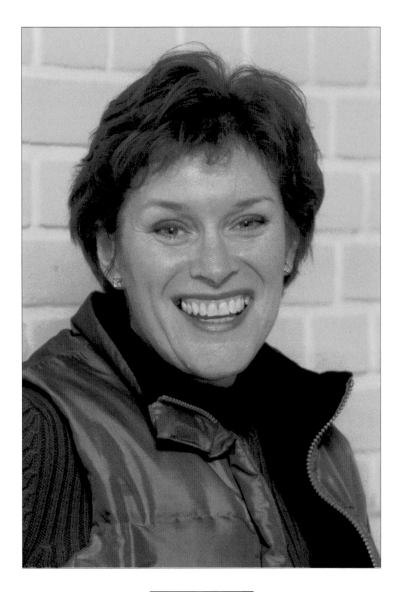

Linda McDonald

They couldn't put an ice-hat on any other hair on my body but my man was certainly turned on by me having no pubic hair and we had a brilliant sex life through it all. Maybe that was heightened by this death-defying crisis we lived through. The box wired up to me certainly gave us some hilarious moments especially during one particularly exciting time when the wire got wrapped around me; I felt like pass the parcel.

We also went on holiday to taste champagne with friends in Rheims and I had only just got the box on. I was in the car when we could hear this beeping noise. Pete thought there was something wrong with his car and we spent ages trying to figure it out, when suddenly I realized it was the battery in my box and I went into a total panic. I had a spare battery with me so I didn't quite fade away!

During treatment I learned to have lots of treats. I had a passion for chips, champagne and Chinese food but my salvation was that I kept working. Just before I got sick I had got a new job working for a US-based foundation helping disadvantaged children around the world and they kept paying me. I worked from home and I went to meetings and I managed to travel too. Going through Heathrow with the box was very funny because I had a letter from the Marsden to explain about the box because we weren't sure if I could go through the security X-ray machine. The chap wanted to see how I was wired up – did they think I had a bomb strapped to me? Well, you have never seen anyone go such an interesting shade of green. He had to go and sit down!

I had worked for children in hospitals before I had cancer, and many of them were sufferers. If a child can be positive and try hard to have fun and play then surely an adult can do it too.

It is now six years since my diagnosis and I have a grand-daughter, a three-year-old princess. I continue to work raising money for charities, and now, with a brilliant volunteer team of business people and experts in children's issues, we are starting our own children's charity – Investors in Children – to harness some of the money being made in stocks and shares and through the Internet. Watch this space!

Linda's tip for surviving treatment

@ Think of the treatment in sections; get through each section so that you have a strong achievement focus.

Linda's book recommendation

@ *Women of Silence: The Emotional Healing of Breast Cancer* by Grace Gawler

Dedicated with thanks to all my friends for their continual love: to Andrew and Jo, my Ma, Nick, Louise, Jason, Vee, Rick Little who kept paying me, and most of all to Steve, who had seen enough of cancer already in his life and walked through this with me, with courage, with love, with fun and lots of tears and laughter

P.S. The most wonderful thing is that my good friend Nick met Liz (one of my nurses at the Marsden) a couple of years ago – they became engaged at midnight on 31 December 1999 and are to marry in the autumn. Happy ending.

DIANA MORAN

Breast cancer turned my world upside down – but from the experience I gained courage, strength and understanding.

Diana Moran, 61, is a television presenter and author. She is best known as BBC *Breakfast Time*'s Green Goddess – the first aerobics teacher to appear on television in England. She has two sons, Tim, 39, and Nick, 37, and four grandchildren, Charlotte, 6, Jessica, 4, Lucy, 2, and James, 6 months. She lives in Surrey.

Diana was diagnosed with breast cancer in 1988, aged 47, at a Well Woman clinic in London. She had a DCIS (ductal carcinoma *in situ*) and opted for a bilateral mastectomy with reconstruction at the Cromwell Hospital, London.

Diana's Story

My breast cancer was discovered by chance twelve years ago when I attended a Well Woman clinic to discuss being a candidate for HRT. It was during one of these visits that I had my first mammogram, at age 47. It was also here that I was told three days later that they had found a suspected tumour. When the news was broken my mind was spinning. I was in tears, the words went in one ear and out the other. I couldn't believe that it had happened to me.

At the time, I was very much in the public arena – I was the first aerobics teacher to appear on television in England as BBC *Breakfast*'s Green Goddess. I had spearheaded fitness awareness in Britain in the 1970s and 1980s and performed in two Royal Command Performances in 1983 and 1984. I was also the author of eight books and numerous fitness videos.

I felt guilty. I thought that I must have done something wrong, especially because I was leading a healthy lifestyle. I worried about how I could face the public with this news but managed to keep it from the media for about six months.

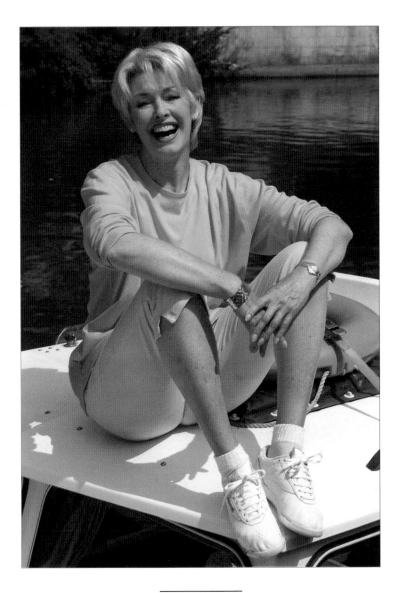

Diana Moran

I desperately wanted and needed privacy at this difficult time in my life, so I checked into the Cromwell Hospital on 2 July 1988 under my maiden name of Dicker. The 7½-hour surgery went well and I was fit and keen to leave the hospital five days later.

As soon as I got home I undressed to take my first bath with trepidation – not knowing how I now looked or how I would feel about myself. To my surprise I was amazed at the reflection I saw in the mirror. As I got out of the bath I felt like a Venus rising from the ocean. I was very happy with my new shape – I'd had immediate reconstruction following the mastectomies. I was so thrilled with how I felt and looked.

I try to stay fit and healthy and think positively. I have an overwhelming sense of joy that I've been given another chance. My life is richer for the experience of breast cancer. I value every day – value life and thank God it's a great day.

In 1993, I took part in 'Le Walk' – a 35-mile charity walk through the Channel Tunnel. For this I received a special medal. I had undergone repeat reconstruction, and a painful divorce, all at the same time and had been feeling physically at my lowest. I'd hit rock bottom. I needed something to focus on. I needed a new goal so I started to get fit.

I met a young man from New Zealand, a cyclist training for the Commonwealth Games. His parents were divorcing and it was affecting him greatly – he was brokenhearted. So we decided to train together in Richmond Park in Surrey. We met in all kinds of weather, snow or ice. I'd walk while he cycled, then we'd sit and chat. We became soulmates. We talked over our problems and cried together and I found my anger was just leaving me. We healed each other. Eventually Chris went back to New Zealand and we haven't seen each other since. But he got me through a very dark patch and trained me up for the walk. This was a turning point in my life and boy did I get fit. The walk was tough going – 35 miles – but by then I had a completely different frame of mind.

This episode helped me put the pieces back together and made me re-evaluate life, and value it. Having cancer has allowed me to show my true strength.

My advice for other women on the rollercoaster that comes with a diagnosis of cancer is: get back in control of your life by asking questions. Find out as much information as possible about the disease, treatment and surgery. Ask as many questions as possible and find someone who has been there to talk to. Talk to the right people. Trust somebody – trust God. I get encouragement and support from women who approach me all the time, to tell me they too have suffered with breast cancer. I also have a role model – my friend Elizabeth, who had breast cancer many years before my diagnosis, but I didn't know. She just gets on with living her life, never complaining.

I have also had the support and love of my family throughout all my ordeals – my two sons, Nick and Tim, and their families, including my four grandchildren, Charlotte, Jessica, Lucy and James, who call me GG – short for Granny Goddess!

Now I concentrate on working hard, which is both a necessity – to keep a roof over my head – and an achievement because I need to have a goal.

My fitness career continues. I am a consultant to the exclusive Le Sport Hotel Spa in St Lucia and La Source in Grenada and I have completed a marathon pantomime season, appearing in 68 performances as the Fairy Godmother in *Cinderella*, alongside Eric Sykes at the Theatre Royal, Windsor.

Very important to me is my involvement in raising public awareness in many charities, including Breakthrough Breast Cancer, Breast Cancer Care, and Cancer Research Campaign to name just a few. For the last three years I have been the Chairman of Stage For Age, a celebrity fundraising charity for Help the Aged, which includes a committee of 70 showbusiness personalities. I have been the president of Osteoporosis Dorset for eight years and I am patron of the Breast Cancer Campaign and the White House Cancer Care Centre in Dudley, East Midlands. I am also the vice-president of Look Good Feel Better, an organization that helps cancer patients regain their dignity and confidence after treatment.

Cancer is a painful experience but from it you can gain courage, strength and understanding. I have gained terrific strength from my experience. Fortune can come and go; good luck can come and go; people can come and go; but if you have good health, you have the most important thing in life. On a rainy day, stuck in traffic and late you can look up to the sky and say, 'It's so good to be alive.'

Diana's tips for surviving treatment

- Ask as many questions as possible.
- Talk to people who have been there.

Diana's prayer recommendation

- 'The Serenity Prayer'

God grant me the serenity
To accept the things I cannot change
The courage to change the things I can
And the wisdom to know the difference.

Dedicated to women throughout the world. With thanks for the support of my family and close friends. They know who they are.

MERCEDES KAY

If you can meet with Triumph and Disaster
And treat those two impostors just the same

'IF', RUDYARD KIPLING

Mercedes Kay, 54, lives in London with her journalist husband John, from whom she has been awarded the OBH – Order of Brilliant Housewife. Mercedes is from Spain and has worked as personal assistant and translator for a leading Spanish politician in Madrid, for the General Manager of Iberia Airlines in London and also for Amnesty International in London.

Mercedes was diagnosed with breast cancer in 1996, aged 50, at the St John and St Elizabeth Hospital, St John's Wood, London. She had a Stage III tumour with two lymph nodes involved. She had a lumpectomy followed by a mastectomy at the St John and St Elizabeth Hospital and six months of chemotherapy at the Royal Free Hospital, Hampstead, London.

Mercedes' Story

This 'story' began in April 1996, while I was on holiday in Cornwall with my husband John and our orange-and-white English Cocker Spaniel Rufus.

As I was having a shower I discovered a lump in my right breast. It was very small and to me it had the shape of a small date. It didn't worry me because seven years previously I'd had two lumps removed from my left breast which both turned out to be benign. But within only two weeks, this latest lump had become very apparent and it had started to hurt.

I went to see my consultant at the Royal Free Hospital, who is one of the top experts on breast cancer in England. He performed a needle biopsy and a week later phoned to say that all was well. But

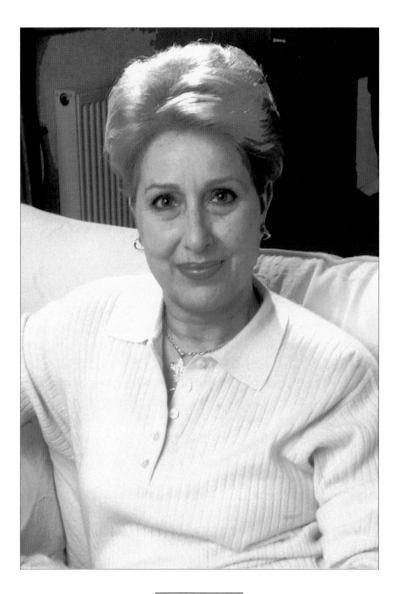

Mercedes Kay

he said that the lump had to be removed and also sent me for an ultrasound scan.

On 13 June, I had a lumpectomy and when the consultant came round to see me in my room that evening he said he had found 'nothing suspicious' but stressed that we would have to wait for the results of the tests on the lump to be sure. Ten days later I had the result of the biopsy. John and I sat in front of the consultant – I was not worried but I noticed that he did not look directly at me. With his eyes looking down at his papers he said, 'I'm afraid it is not good news.'

He went on but I just could not understand what he was talking about. So I asked him, 'Do you mean I have cancer?' and he said yes. After my initial reaction of utter disbelief and bewilderment, I felt very sad and frightened – sheer terror in fact – and I thought I had reached the end of my life. I thought, am I going to die? The following morning before going to work, John – who has a very outgoing personality and is a very positive and optimistic person – sat by me and cried inconsolably. It was the first and only time I have ever seen him crying. He told me that he felt 'so sorry' for me. That really shook me and I thought I had been given a second chance and in no way was I going to waste it! The thought of 'leaving him' encouraged me to fight with all my strength. I was prepared to go through everything modern science had to offer me in order to get cured. Everything was going to be all right.

I started a six-month course of chemotherapy at the Royal Free at the beginning of August and it lasted until the end of January 1997. I kept a diary and, although the first eight weeks were depressing, very soon I developed a kind of 'visual' friendship with other women suffering adversity and misfortune.

One extract from my diary reads: 'There is a kind of complicity between us. We understand each other with our eyes. It is extremely moving to see young mothers receiving chemo with their children beside them. There are women of all ages – some have been on chemo for a very long time and they are alive and kicking and joking! That is what is motivating me!'

I started to believe that cancer was not a death sentence, that it was a myth that cancer was incurable. But I also felt isolated because I realized that both my family and some of my friends did not know what to say to me. Some even stopped phoning me altogether – I believe that they were frightened themselves. When all the words from the outside world seemed quite superfluous, one of the women receiving chemo said to me, 'You have to learn to treat cancer as any other illness.' What a good tip that was. These other women were a great inspiration to me.

Before the chemo, John and I went out to buy a wig and also two different types of shampoo for it. I never had to use it – but I still keep it because I am superstitious. My hair went a bit thin, but my eyebrows and much-admired eyelashes disappeared. However, I still wore makeup and tried to look my best. A bit of lipstick and a good pair of earrings worked wonders! I also went out every day – except once when I felt very sick after having a Chinese takeaway.

At the end of the chemo, we went to see the consultant who said that we could 'take a chance' and leave the right breast as it was. But when he said that there would be a 30 per cent chance of the cancer returning to the right breast, I did not hesitate for a second and opted for the radical mastectomy. I am now on tamoxifen and go for check-ups every four months – the consultant said that I could go every six months but I prefer to go more frequently for my own peace of mind. Now I realize that still there are some misunderstandings about cancer. Betty Westgate, MBE (Founder and President of Breast Cancer Care), says that 'many thought that cancer was a modern disease and were most surprised to hear that there is evidence of it existing in the times of the ancient Egyptian Pharaohs'. I used to think that breast cancer was a type of punishment from God for youthful misdeeds and consequently felt guilty – what a load of 'B'.

Now, nearly four years after I found the lump, I can see that my life has changed . . . for the better. I feel fulfilled and privileged to be able to love life so intensely. I used to have a phobia about spiders – they came out of my fireplace in all sizes and I stamped on them. Not any more. I let them pass by me . . . life is too precious. In the last three years I have made many new good friends in London and I enjoy their company, and that of my loved ones, better than ever before. In short,

I'm delighting in life. I've become more creative, understanding, tolerant, wiser and, above all, a better person.

What are my ambitions now? Live, live, live. And to be with the people and things I love, including my dog, Rufus. I find true pleasure in nature (my walks with Rufus and friends, the garden, and all sorts of creatures) and I'm very proud of my husband John who supported me and helped me before, during, and after my operations and chemotherapy.

Talking and writing about it all is very good therapy which is why I felt honoured and happy when I was approached to write my story for this book. In a nutshell, family and friends should not be afraid of talking to cancer sufferers.

Mercedes' tip for surviving treatment

🌳 Don't be frightened – it's going to be all right.

Mercedes' music recommendation

🌳 Dvorak's 'New World' Symphony (No. 9)

Dedicated to my beloved husband John

CATHERINE WALKER

En toi, garde un immense amour!
Keep your heart full of love!

Catherine Walker, 55, is one of Britain's leading fashion designers. Few people knew of her extraordinary relationship with her client of sixteen years, Diana, Princess of Wales, whose image Catherine is now generally regarded as having created. In 1990 and 1991, Catherine won the BFC's Designer of the Year award for couture and glamour. She is from France and lives in London with her husband. She has two daughters, Naomi, 29, and Marianne, 27.

Catherine was diagnosed with breast cancer in 1995, aged 50, at a London clinic. She had a lumpectomy and 26 sessions of radiotherapy at the Cromwell Hospital, London.

Catherine's Story

On 27 August 1975 my husband, John, died in a tragic accident while we were on holiday in France, leaving me a widow with two baby daughters. My husband was 32 years old and the abruptness of his death left many unresolved emotions both in his family and in mine. I mention this because I believe it may have been the main reason why I later developed cancer. Of course I cannot prove the connection and anyone who relies only on scientific evidence would mock the idea.

Twenty years later, together with my second husband and business partner, I was hard at work in a successful business I had started primarily to deal with the grief of widowhood. However, all was not well. I had started to suffer rather severe symptoms of menopause, and so I visited my gynaecologist who prescribed Hormone Replacement Therapy (HRT). I showed him a lump in my left breast which he said was nothing. A year later the lump had grown and it was cancer.

Today, as I write this, it is exactly five years past that first diagnosis and I have learned much about this terrifying disease, my body and my lifestyle both professional and private. I should explain that my experience is not typical and I would not offer it as a guide to others. My body is so sensitive that it has stretched the credibility of most doctors I have ever met.

When I was first diagnosed, the shock was of course devastating and questions crowded into my mind. How did it happen? What was going to happen to me? How could I help myself? I felt lost as if I didn't even know the questions let alone the answers. I started reading books on the subject and asking lots of questions, and as a result I became aware of the following.

Firstly, I did not 'catch' cancer. It was part of me and I had allowed it to grow. Doctors I have spoken to believe that we all have cancer cells in us but they do not grow if we – or more specifically our immune systems – are strong enough to resist them. Secondly, rather than just focusing on cancer, I was better off focusing on how I was going to be in ten years' time and imagining myself as a healthier and stronger person than ever before. Thirdly, because my cancer was not irreversibly advanced I could decide to some extent what was going to happen to me.

My cancer was a lump which measured 1.2cm in diameter. I had radiotherapy treatment – my oncologist did not offer me chemo-therapy because he knew that I was not going to accept it in any case, and the decision was borderline. I decided against tamoxifen. This is a controversial decision and I was only able to do this with the help of my doctors who wisely acknowledged the sensitivity of my body and other factors, and allowed me to make the final choice.

I made a list of the adjunctive treatments about which I wanted to enquire. I saw a wonderful acupuncturist throughout my treatment and indeed continue to do so today – on the adjunctive side I am convinced he saved my life. There are nutritionists who specialize in fighting cancer through diet and after a few mishaps (sensitivity again) I started a diet which most people would find a little daunting. I consulted a hormone specialist as my cancer was hormone-dependent and I was not taking tamoxifen. Following my operation, which included surgery under the arm, I found I had a frozen shoulder and later sciatica. I found both Alexander technique and Qigong invaluable then and have ever since. I now wonder whether there is a connection between cancer, frozen shoulder, sciatica and unresolved emotions. I recently started to see a counsellor and find his help extremely valuable.

I did all these things with the support of my family, friends, clients and staff. I cherished the little gifts I was given by those who loved me: flowers, paper cranes, front-opening shirts that you can easily take off, etc. Above all I had the exquisite support of my husband who was at my bedside every moment I was awake in hospital for my lumpectomy, accompanied me on every one of my 26 radiotherapy treatments, and even now accompanies me on every check-up visit.

Cancer has brought me the benefit of appreciating my body rather than, as I have done all my life, feeling apologetic and awkward about its sensitivity. I listen to my body because it tells me things a more robust body would overlook. My advice to any woman who has just been diagnosed with breast cancer is to listen to your body and trust your instinct in your choice of treatment, whether conventional, alternative or both. Keep listening to any changes that might occur in your body. It is an ongoing process, and for me it has taught me a lifetime's lesson.

I have changed my way of working, I do fewer hours, I take a step at a time and try to enjoy it to the maximum. I am more tender towards myself. I spend more time in the country walking and appreciating nature. Cancer has caused me to notice things – who I love and who loves me, what I should care about and not care about. The fashion world can be very silly and things that used to bother me now simply pass over my head. I am proud that I have no bitterness in me and I am often reminded of a poem my great-uncle Achile, a wonderful character with a long white beard, wrote for me about love. I read it whenever I need to remember that the most important thing is to be happy with my husband and, of course, our two daughters to whom I dedicate this piece because they are women. I hope they cherish their femininity and do not stretch themselves too

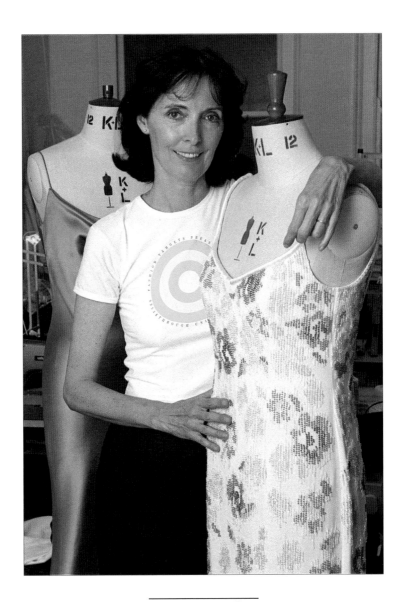

Catherine Walker

hard as I might have done. Women are wonderful, fragile creatures, the centre of the family and therefore society.

> *Petite princesse lointaine,*
> *tu rêves de bouquets de fleurs*
> *de sonorités, de couleurs,*
> *de mer bleue et de vastes plaines . . .*
> *Tandis qu'aux heures incertaines*
> *dans le soir gris tombent nos pleurs,*
> *tu ne rêves que de bonheurs;*
> *comment les saisir à mains pleines.*
> *Comment les conserver? Surtout,*
> *comment garder, suprême atout*
> *l'enthousiasme et la jeunesse?*
> *Ah! pour que nulle heure, des jours*
> *à venir, jamais ne te blesse:*
> *En toi, garde un immense amour!*

This is my translation into English:

> *Little Princess far away,*
> *you dream of flower bouquets,*
> *of sounds, of colours,*
> *of blue seas, of vast plains . . .*
>
> *While during the uncertain grey hours*
> *of evening our tears fall,*
> *you dream only of happiness*
> *and how to seize it with open hands.*
>
> *How do you cherish it? Most of all,*
> *how do you keep it, this supreme asset of*
> *enthusiasm and youth?*
>
> *Ah! So that no hour of any day*
> *ever comes to hurt you,*
> *keep your heart full of love!*
> ACHILE SEVIN, AIX-EN-PROVENCE, JUNE 1960

Catherine's tips for surviving treatment

- Meditation
- Acupuncture
- Healthy diet
- Alexander technique
- Qigong

Catherine's book recommendation

- *Alternative Medicine: The Definitive Guide To Cancer* by W. John Diamond et al.

Dedicated to Naomi and Marianne

GWYNETH DORRICOTT

There is a law in life: when one door closes to us another one opens.
ANDRÉ GIDE

Gwyneth Dorricott, 63, has worked with children for 26 years, teaching those with special needs and setting up programmes for Special Needs pupils. She has owned her own shop selling handpainted leisurewear, which she makes herself and also exhibits throughout the UK. She has a daughter, Jacqui, aged 35, and a son, Paul, aged 33. She lives in Seaford, East Sussex.

Gwyneth was diagnosed with breast cancer in 1990, aged 52, at a routine screening of women over 50, at the Coventry and Warwickshire Hospital. She had a mastectomy and axillary clearance at the Hospital of St Cross, Rugby, followed by a month of radiotherapy at the Walsgrave Hospital, Coventry.

Gwyneth's Story

After a rewarding lifetime in education, I was working with Special Needs children in Coventry, teaching in several schools and setting up programmes in mainstream schools for children with learning difficulties.

Life was always hectic: taking groups of children camping in Wales by minibus, day trips to a farm, trips to visit the cathedral or going swimming for the afternoon – all spare time was booked. The emphasis on practical experience was vital to aid the learning programme.

In 1989 I entered the Coventry Walkathon, walking 20 miles sponsored for charity. Another week I went with colleagues to Snowdonia to prepare for a visit by some of our children to an outdoor-pursuits centre. We climbed Snowdon, took canoes out to

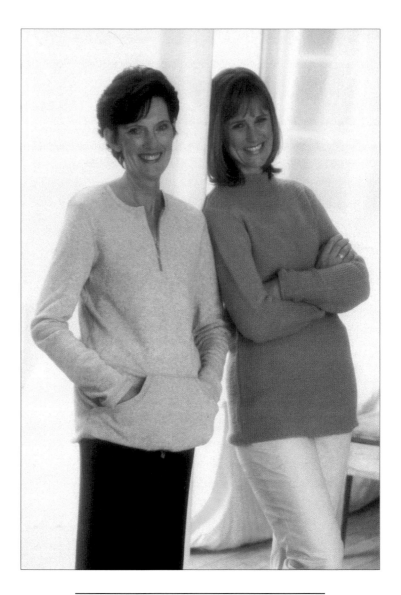

Gwyneth Dorricott with daughter Jacqui

sea and generally tried out the centre which was excellent for city youngsters.

Another half-term, my son and I took camping gear in the minibus and followed our two deputy headteachers on their sponsored cycle coast to coast, St Bees to Whitby.

Suddenly, following a routine X-ray for women over 50, I was diagnosed with breast cancer and within a fortnight was rushed from classroom to hospital. My life was to change drastically.

I was well supported by a lovely daughter and dear son, family and friends; 'get well' cards, flowers and phone calls came daily. The most important phone call came from Gill, a close friend and colleague, the deputy headteacher at my school. She had lost a member of her family through cancer and asked which specialist I was being treated by. When I told her she said, 'You are going to be all right, Gwyneth. Your consultant is one of the finest in Britain.' She was so right. At the breast clinic the care was kind and personal, the sympathy comforting and the treatment so efficient. I was glad to be able to entrust my care to the experts.

After having a mastectomy I found that people were setting me goals to work on! My brother rang and said, 'I'm expecting you in Tenerife in nine weeks' time.' After constant check-ups and feeling a little shaky – but with a couple of sessions with the breast-care nurse to set me up with a comfy bra – I was on the plane to Tenerife! As I left I heard my brave daughter say, 'Mum, when you're well, I'm taking you away anywhere in the world that you want to go.' There was no chance to feel sorry for myself – only to fight on and get ready for the adventure of a lifetime.

In January 1991, we left Heathrow with rucksacks, bound for Thailand. Most of my clothes were in Jacqui's bag. We arrived in Bangkok to see palaces, Buddhas and a variety of lovely, smiling faces. We travelled on minibus, tuk-tuks, trains, elephants, rickshaws and boats through an amazing country. Through Chiang Mai to the Golden Triangle overlooking Burma; Vietnam, the Mekong to the North; then south to the lovely coast of Hua Hin and Phuket, spending a week in a beach bungalow on Phi Phi Ko Island. It was idyllic.

Jacqui had taken nearly three months out of her profession to set me on my feet again, ready for the further challenges life has to offer. As Jacqui continuously devotes herself to others' happiness, it's impossible to thank her, but I hope that the fact that I am here, ten years on, and love her dearly, may suffice for the time being.

From Phi Phi and Phuket, I flew to join my brother in Singapore where he had booked a beautiful hotel room for me, where an orchid was laid on my pillow each night. I took a taxi to see the gem factories and a boat to tour the harbour. Two days later we flew back to Hua Hin and Bangkok ready for the flight home. How different my life had become.

As my special subject in my profession had always been art, my head was full of the memories: of glittering colours, dazzling patterns and the beauty of Thailand. I set about decorating a few T-shirts with some glitter paint. Before long and with my friends' encouragement, I had a collection – silver dolphins and gold and glittery abstracts were ready for a trial run at a local craft fair. Many more shows followed and eventually I set up shop with a partner for three years. Now I am 62 and retired – almost!

Last year, I entered a competition run by one of our favourite ladieswear shops – and won. My daughter and I found ourselves being entertained in London and treated to a makeover. We were so spoilt. At a studio in central London we were treated like royalty, having our makeup and hair done, then being photographed by a top fashion photographer, wearing the latest lovely clothes. At the end of the day I was told I could have a part-time job if I wanted!

Life is so precious and I feel so lucky to have experienced the past ten years. My daughter and son have been such a comfort and support, my brother and family too. I am proud to have worked with children for 26 years, and especially to have worked with the children in two schools in Coventry, where the staff were dedicated professionals – a 'special breed' working tirelessly as a team to educate those with learning difficulties. I was fortunate that their caring support was extended to me in my time of need.

I feel that through adversity, life acquires another dimension, an urgency to appreciate. I am much more philosophical now, priorities change and I value the really important issues so much more. My advice to someone who is newly faced with breast cancer is to gratefully take hold of the many hands that will be offered to you and always look forward to tomorrow.

Gwyneth's tip for surviving treatment

✿ Find out about your specialist as far as possible and feel happy that you have the best possible attention.

Gwyneth's book recommendation

✿ *Springs of Hope: Book of Sayings*

Dedicated to Mr T. Alan Waterworth, FRCS, Consultant Surgeon, a dedicated specialist in the fight against breast cancer, highly regarded by his many patients

CARLY SIMON

It's the soul and the spirit that are either beautiful or not . . . If anyone loves me, I want it to be for my natural self.

Carly Simon, 55, is a singer who is best known for her seventies hits 'You're So Vain' and 'Nobody Does It Better' as well as the film *Heartburn*'s theme tune 'Coming Around Again'. She was married to singer James Taylor, who is the father of her two children, Sally, 26 and Ben, 23. She lives in New York with her husband, novelist Jim Hart.

Carly was diagnosed with breast cancer in 1997, aged 52. She had a lumpectomy followed by chemotherapy.

Carly's Story

I feel stronger and more vital than ever. It takes some time to get used to the fear of having cancer but I always thought of myself as a warrior. When you actually have a battle it's better than when you don't know who to fight.

I've visited some women who are so much worse off. My heart breaks for them. This disease is practically an epidemic. We need a lot more money for research. There's a feeling that if this was a man's disease it would have been licked already.

During my operation they got everything and the prognosis was good so my doctor gave me the option of whether to have chemotherapy. I decided to play it safe – and the treatments were only every three weeks. I thought I would lose my hair so I bought lots of wigs. I never had to wear them.

I don't want to be singled out but the idea of somebody stopping me in the street to say 'I'm sorry' is a kind of downer. Then I have to comfort them. The less explaining I have to do the more energy I have to take care of myself.

It sounds weird to say but it feels like a gift. I'm feeling so creative. I've hardly ever had a period where I've been so fruitful writing songs. I don't know whether it's a side-effect. Anything that's scary like this reminds you how precious life is.

Dedicated to Linda McCartney

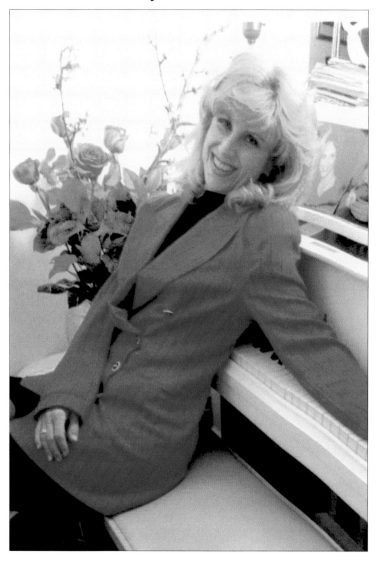

Carly Simon

SHIRLEY HARWOOD

Don't let your cancer be the winner, you can beat it.

Shirley Harwood, 65, lives in Jersey with her husband Dennis. She retired in 1994 as Head of Midwifery Services at the Jersey General Hospital. She has three sons, Andrew, 38, Richard, 36, and Phillip, who unfortunately died at two days old, and a granddaughter, Emma, 7.

Shirley was diagnosed with breast cancer in 1995, aged 59, at the Jersey General Hospital. She had a mastectomy and axillary clearance at the London Bridge Hospital and six weeks of radiotherapy at the Royal South Hampshire Hospital, Southampton.

Shirley's Story

I cannot recall my thoughts during the short walk from the hospital to my husband's office in May 1995 except, how was I going to explain to my beloved Den (a definite boob man), whom I had repeatedly reassured over the last few months that the lump in my breast was nothing, that it was, in fact, something? When he came out of his office, I immediately burst into tears, apologizing for having breast cancer and needing a mastectomy. He was wonderful and we went to Liberation Square and sat and talked through this bombshell.

A week after my diagnosis, I was at the London Bridge Hospital, accompanied by my son Andrew, awaiting my mastectomy. On the day of my surgery I was not allowed to eat or drink anything after 10 a.m. so we rose early that morning and 'the condemned woman ate a hearty breakfast'!

The surgery was at 6 p.m. and I don't recall anything further until later that evening when I awoke to find my chest tightly bandaged and a drain in my left side. I slept quite well and the following morning was able to wash myself and make myself presentable for the arrival of Den and our younger son Richard. They were both delighted to see how well I looked and felt.

A week later, on the following Saturday, the consultant suggested I go out for a walk despite still having a drain *in situ* complete with drainage bottle! When this was suggested I felt very anxious. I didn't want to get dressed. I felt fine about my missing breast while wearing my night-dress and dressing-gown but found it difficult to visualize being dressed in clothes I'd worn when I was 'normal'. We left it until the following day when I dressed in the clothes I'd arrived in, although I felt it was glaringly obvious to everyone that I'd had a mastectomy. I was assured that with a cardigan around my shoulders, to hide the drainage system, you couldn't tell at all.

It was a beautiful day so we walked over London Bridge and sat on the Embankment watching the world go by. As my wardrobe consisted of just one outfit, the following day we took a taxi to Marks and Spencer (I being never one to miss an opportunity to shop) and purchased skirts, tops and scarves – the latter fortunately in fashion and suggested by the nurses, to tie and hang down the 'missing side'. This proved to be a great morale-booster and we continued to enjoy sunny days on the Embankment including a visit to the Tower of London. Ten days after my surgery Den and I returned to Jersey.

The consultant did not feel it was necessary for me to have chemotherapy but I did need to have radiotherapy for six weeks. Unfortunately, this treatment is not available in the Channel Islands so once again it meant going to the mainland. I opted for the hospital in Southampton which is the centre normally used by Channel Island residents. This proved to be the most difficult part of my treatment – not the treatment itself but the loneliness of being away from the family. I spoke to them two or three times a day and went home every weekend but I still recall this period as being horrendous.

My treatment started in July and finished at the beginning of September. As a surprise, Den booked us a two-week holiday in Mauritius at the end of September. The holiday was wonderful, just what we both needed to recharge our batteries. We spent the days walking, reading, sleeping and, best of all, swimming in the sea.

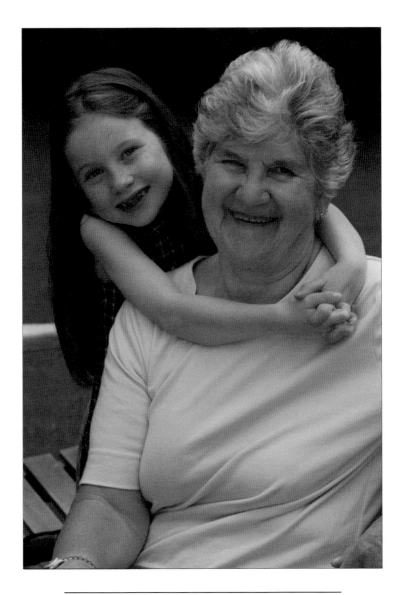

Shirley Harwood with granddaughter Emma

After our return home, life got back to normal quickly – Den went back to work, I returned to my daily swimming sessions, seeing Emma, my granddaughter, meeting friends and making trips to London for my check-ups. However, by the end of October I had started to feel very down. I didn't feel I was going anywhere or had anything to look forward to. Then one day I received a phone call from one of my ex-colleagues, saying that she desperately needed help with her aquanatal classes and that if I was interested, there was a course being run in London on 18 and 19 November. The course was very intensive and involved classroom and pool work so I was constantly in and out of the water. Fortunately, by this time I had purchased a couple of swimming prostheses. I successfully completed the course and returned to Jersey to organize and conduct three aquanatal classes per week – working in the pool and poolside. I loved it, I was back in my favourite occupation, working with pregnant ladies, helping them through their labours and seeing the end product!

Although I appeared to have accepted my loss – when I was up and dressed I didn't look any different to anyone else – bedtimes were a constant reminder that I had had cancer. My husband had been wonderful and accepted my changed body from day one and our sex life was as good as ever, but whenever I turned over in bed I was reminded that I'd had breast cancer.

Although I had enquired prior to my mastectomy about immediate reconstruction, my consultant said he preferred to wait until all treatment was completed. It was now that I began to seriously consider reconstruction. My husband thought it was totally unnecessary, that I'd 'been through enough' but if it was what I wanted, he would support me. By this time, we had a consultant in Jersey doing breast reconstruction with superb results, so I made an appointment to see him and as a result I underwent a TRAM reconstruction in February 1997, with an excellent outcome.

After that it was as if the mastectomy had never happened. My husband joined me in retirement two years ago and life is wonderful. We take frequent trips to London to see my family and have been on many exotic holidays.

I keep very active and continue to swim 40 lengths a day. Den and I love to walk the dogs and work in our garden. We are also renovating our bungalow and have completed many DIY projects in the house, including putting in new floors and bathrooms and redecorating. I also love having my granddaughter Emma come to stay in the school holidays.

I have recently had my five-year check-up when I received the usual comment – 10 out of 10!

May 1996. Scene: hotel room with Papa, Grandma and Emma age 2½ years. Grandma in the bathroom when Emma walks in.

'Grandma, you've only got one. Mummy's got two, Daddy's got two, Papa's got two and I've got two but you've only got one.' *Grandma gives simple explanation of how that one was poorly and had to be taken away.*

May 1997. Scene: local swimming-pool changing room, very proud Grandma (now I have two) and Emma.

'Grandma, you've only got one. Mummy's got two, Daddy's got two, Papa's got two and I've got two but you've only got one.' *Indignant Grandma*: 'I've got two now.' *Exasperated Emma*: 'No, Grandma, those [*pointing to the nipple*]; you've only got one.' At this stage, nipple reconstruction was scheduled for June 1997.

GRANDMA NOW HAS TWO.

Shirley's tip for surviving treatment

🌱 Think positively; don't let your cancer be the winner, you can beat it.

Shirley's book recommendations

🌱 *A Woman's Decision* by Karen Berger and John Bostock III, MD
🌱 *Living Beyond Breast Cancer: A Survivor's Guide* by Marisa C. Weis, MD, and Ellen Weis

Dedicated to my family and friends

PART
2
RESOURCE
GUIDE

THE ROYAL MARSDEN NHS TRUST

RECENT IMPROVEMENTS IN CANCER MEDICINE

IAN E. SMITH, MD, FRCP, FRCPE
PROFESSOR OF CANCER MEDICINE
ROYAL MARSDEN HOSPITAL AND INSTITUTE OF CANCER RESEARCH

Breast cancer touches nearly everyone in one way or another, either directly or through family and friends. More than 30,000 women develop breast cancer every year in the UK and the number is rising. Despite this, there is good news. For the first time ever, the death rate is falling and today there are more breast cancer survivors than ever before. Last year, for example, there were more than 1,500 fewer deaths in the UK than ten years ago.

The reason for this can be summed up in one word – teamwork. Today, as never before, surgeons, physicians with their medical treatments, radiotherapists, pathologists and nurse specialists are working together from the moment each patient first enters the clinic, to try to eradicate every last breast cancer cell from the body.

Understanding breast cancer

For a long time breast cancer was considered to be a localized disease which spread slowly through the breast until it reached the glands in the armpit (or axilla), which were seen as a gateway or barrier to the rest of the body. Bloodstream spread to other parts of the body was believed to be only a late event. The mainstay of treatment was therefore major surgery and in particular radical mastectomy. Gradually it became apparent that surgery alone, however extensive, did not cure the majority of patients. The concept was wrong.

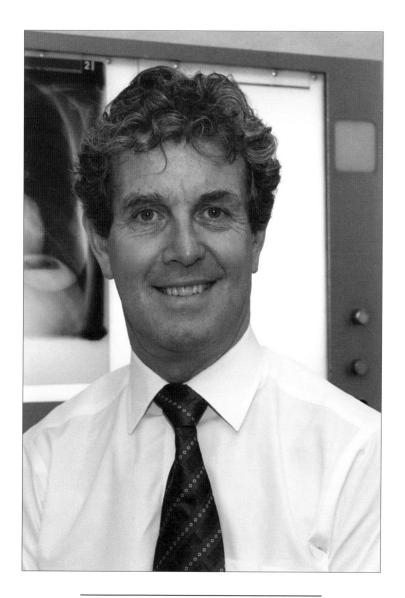

Professor Ian Smith, MD, FRCP, FRCPE

It is now understood that the first breast cancer cells probably develop several years before the cancer is detected and in most patients some cancer cells escape into the bloodstream and spread to other parts of the body early on, well before the patient first becomes aware of a lump in the breast. Surgery alone cannot correct this problem.

Adjuvant medical therapy

This term refers to drug treatment given at the same time as surgery, to kill off microscopic cancer cells elsewhere in the body, and its development is the main reason why the breast cancer death rate is at last falling. There are two main kinds of treatment.

The first includes a drug called tamoxifen. This drug, a British discovery, has been used to treat millions of women worldwide. In my view, it is quite simply the most successful anti-cancer drug ever, in terms of lives saved and lack of serious side-effects. Many (but not all) breast cancers are stimulated by the female hormone oestrogen, and tamoxifen blocks this effect without blocking the natural beneficial effects of oestrogen; these include protection against osteoporosis (bone thinning) and heart attacks. Trials throughout the world have confirmed that adjuvant tamoxifen decreases the risk of breast cancer recurring after surgery, in patients whose cancers have a biological marker called oestrogen receptor. Current evidence suggests that it works best if given for around five years and it seems to be particularly beneficial in older women. As an added bonus, tamoxifen also reduces the risk of another cancer developing in the opposite breast. Nothing is perfect, however, and tamoxifen's main problem is that it slightly increases the risk of cancer of the womb.

The second form of adjuvant therapy involves chemotherapy. There are many different forms of this but all of them involve drugs specifically designed to kill cancer cells directly. Chemotherapy is usually given by a short running drip once every three weeks or so for around six courses. Unfortunately, chemotherapy can have short-term, unpleasant side-effects which include tiredness, nausea and, sometimes, hair loss (which always recovers). Despite this, chemotherapy, like tamoxifen, decreases the risk of breast cancer coming back after surgery, particularly in younger women. In the past, chemotherapy was used only in high-risk patients with aggressive forms of breast cancer. More recently, it has become clear that chemotherapy can reduce the risk of recurrence still further even in patients with a relatively good outlook anyway.

The choice of adjuvant therapy for the individual patient depends on many factors including the grade of cancer (i.e., what it looks like under the microscope), whether the axillary glands are involved or not, the size of the cancer and whether it has oestrogen receptors or not (so-called receptor positive.) For many women the best choice is both chemotherapy and tamoxifen.

Radiotherapy

Radiotherapy involves the use of powerful X-rays to destroy any residual cancer cells left behind in the breast, the chest wall or the glands after surgery. It is usually given in short daily treatments for several weeks. Its main role is to prevent recurrence in these local areas, but recent trials have shown that it also improves the survival chances in some patients.

New drugs

There is no other cancer in which so many promising new drugs have appeared over the last few years and breast cancer specialists are currently facing the challenge of how best to use these to cut down deaths still further. These new drugs include the following:

Tamoxifen-like drugs called SERMs (selective estrogen receptor modifiers) are being developed which are active against breast cancer but without the risk of womb cancer and which also have all the beneficial effects of oestrogens. Recently progress has also been made with a new class of drugs called aromatase inhibitors (e.g., Arimidex, letrozole) which block the production of oestrogens and control breast cancer growth with only minimal side-effects. Likewise, a new generation of so-called pure anti-oestrogens are becoming available which may be more effective and longer-lasting than tamoxifen itself.

Several powerful new chemotherapy drugs have also emerged in the last few years, including taxotere (not to be confused with tamoxifen), taxol and navelbine, and there is already evidence that these may be better than our older agents. Other similar drugs are on the horizon with the promise of fewer side-effects, and some of these are going to be available as tablets rather than by injection. Bone is a particular target for breast cancer spread; recently a new class of compounds called biphosphonates (clodronate, pamidronate) has been discovered which specifically protect the bones from attack by breast cancer cells, and trials are under way to see if these can prevent recurrence in bone.

Finally, a more 'natural' form of treatment using a specifically designed antibody therapy (Herceptin) has just been developed which targets a protein called HER2 on the cell surface of some aggressive forms of breast cancer. This has already achieved regressions in some patients with very advanced disease, and wide-scale trials will soon start in early disease, to try to increase cure rates.

High-risk women

We don't really understand what causes breast cancer in most women but the disease is much commoner in the affluent West than in the Third World. Diet and delayed onset of childbearing are probably part of the explanation. In a small minority of women (say 5–10 per cent) breast cancer appears to run strongly in families and is genetically inherited. Two so-called breast cancer genes, BRCA1 and BRCA2, have already been identified and it is likely that others will be found. Genetic testing is now available to identify potential carriers of these abnormal genes, but it is important to remember that in the great majority of patients breast cancer is sporadic; that is, the disease is not inherited but arises 'out of the blue' without any obvious cause.

Breast cancer prevention

The female hormone oestrogen is in some way responsible for causing breast cancer. This has led to trials of the oestrogen-blocking drug tamoxifen in high-risk women to see if breast cancer can be prevented. So far results from different trials are conflicting but it seems likely that tamoxifen may prevent breast cancer at least in some groups of women. New trials are now under way with tamoxifen-like drugs that may have less long-term risk (SERMs, as described above) and also with natural food additives such as red clover extract. I think it is likely that breast cancer prevention will become a major new success story in a few years' time.

Conclusions

For the first time, real progress is being made in the treatment of breast cancer. At last we are beginning to understand the underlying biology of the disease, we have learned how to combine surgical with medical treatments, and a whole range of new drugs is being developed. Breast cancer is still one of the biggest challenges facing modern medicine, but the future looks much brighter than the past.

BREAST AWARENESS

Every woman, no matter what age, should become breast aware.

Check your breasts regularly, about once a month – more frequently might mean subtle changes go unnoticed.

Breast awareness is about learning how your breasts feel and knowing what is normal for you. There is no need to follow any particular routine, just be aware of any changes in your breast. Do this by looking and feeling in any way you feel most comfortable – the bath, shower, when dressing, standing or lying down.

Any changes that occur can be more easily detected when you are familiar with how your breasts normally look and feel.

Changes to look out for:

- A change in the outline, shape or size of the breast, especially caused by arm movements, or by lifting the breasts. Any puckering or dimpling of the skin.

- Lumps, thickening or bumpy areas in one breast or armpit that seem to be different from the same part of the other breast and armpit, especially if new.

- Nipple discharge that is new; bleeding or moist reddish areas that don't heal easily; any change in nipple position; or a rash around the nipple.

- New or persistent pain or tenderness within the breast.

- New veins that stand out, particularly on one breast and not the other.

- Any changes that you find that are new to you should be checked out by your GP.

- Remember that 9 out of 10 lumps or changes are harmless and are not cancer. However, it is important to have a GP check anything unusual, as early detection of any cancer greatly increases one's chance of survival.

Resources (for details see Recommended Books)
Breast Awareness (Breakthrough)
Everything You Need to Know About Breast Awareness (Royal Marsden)

DIAGNOSIS AND TREATMENTS

Early diagnosis of cancer is the key to survival. With that in mind women should regularly check their breasts for lumps – especially younger women who tend to fall through the safety net of breast screening. They should not be worried if they find a lump because 9 out of 10 breast lumps are not cancerous – they are benign. But they should seek advice from their GPs. The lump may be a fluid-filled cyst or a fibroadenoma (an overgrowth of fibrous tissue), each of which can be easily treated.

Here is a list of testing procedures that you may follow, if you discover a lump, before you receive a diagnosis.

Breast screening

As breast cancer is more common in post-menopausal women, a screening programme has been set up in the UK inviting women between the ages of 50 and 64 to regularly attend breast clinics for mammograms.

Women over the age of 65 may attend any clinic without an invitation but with an appointment. Women who have a family history of breast cancer may be offered screening or other tests at an earlier age.

Women under 50 who are concerned about changes in their breasts should consult with their GP, as should all other women who are between clinic visits. Early detection is vital.

Mammograms

A mammogram is an X-ray of the breast tissue. It may show changes in your breasts before they are felt or noticed by you or your doctor.

To be X-rayed, your breasts will be pressed firmly between two pieces of plastic. The mammogram may be uncomfortable for some women but it only takes a few minutes.

Ultrasound scan

An ultrasound scan uses sound waves to build up a picture of your breasts. It can determine the difference between a solid lump and a fluid-filled cyst. It is very painless and is similar to the scanning of a baby during pregnancy.

For the ultrasound scan to be taken, a gel is spread over your breasts and a sensor is lightly moved across the skin.

Aspiration for cytology

Either a fine needle or a syringe is used to take a sample of cells from the lump. The needle or syringe is inserted into the lump and a few cells are drawn up and then examined under a microscope in the laboratory (cytology).

This test is very quick and performed without a local anaesthetic, either in the clinic or in hospital.

Biopsy

A biopsy is a procedure whereby a sample of breast tissue is removed to be examined under the microscope in a laboratory.

A tru-cut biopsy is where a core of tissue is removed, and may be performed in an outpatient clinic using a local anaesthetic. You may feel some discomfort and pressure during this biopsy.

Other biopsies may require general anaesthetic and admittance to hospital for the day or overnight. Your general health will be checked before the operation, with chest X-rays and blood tests.

If, on a mammogram, an abnormality is spotted which is difficult for the doctor to feel, the area is localized before the operation. This requires insertion of a fine wire into the lump in the breast, under local anaesthetic, with the guidance of the mammogram X-rays and ultrasound. This pinpoints the area of tissue that should be removed. The wire is then removed during the operation.

After the operation, a drain from the incision is left in place to remove any excess fluid and blood produced by the biopsy. This is usually removed the following day, before you leave the hospital.

Determining the right surgery

If you receive a diagnosis of breast cancer, a lot of factors come into play in determining the best course of surgery you should have and whether pre- and post-operative chemotherapy and radiotherapy are also required. The results of a series of tests performed on the biopsy, together with the location and size of the malignant tumour and whether it is invasive or *in situ*, will indicate which surgery is best for you.

If the tumour is considered inoperable owing to its size, a course of radiotherapy and/or chemotherapy may be offered initially, to shrink the tumour down to a size where it can be removed during surgery.

Ductal carcinoma *in situ* (DCIS)

DCIS is the earliest stage of breast cancer which cannot normally be felt, therefore it only shows up on a mammogram as calcifications – white calcium deposits. It is a non-invasive cancer that is confined to the breast duct and has not spread within the breast tissue or outside it.

If DCIS is found extensively throughout the breast then a mastectomy may be required. For a small area of DCIS found and removed at biopsy, a wide local excision (lumpectomy) may be all that is required, followed by radiotherapy.

Invasive carcinoma

If the malignant tumour cells have started to infiltrate the surrounding breast tissue, including the blood and lymph supply, the tumour is considered invasive. Lumpectomies or mastectomies are performed on this type of cancer, together with chemotherapy and radiotherapy, to kill off any microscopic cells that have travelled around the body to other sites, that may form secondary or metastatic tumours. The first area checked for cancer spread outside the breast is the axillary (underarm) lymph nodes. Other common secondary tumour sites for breast cancer include bone, lungs and liver.

Types of surgery

Lumpectomy

The surgery that removes the tumour and some of the surrounding normal tissue is known as a lumpectomy. It is also known as a wide local excision, segmentectomy, partial or segmental mastectomy or quadrantectomy. Lymph nodes may or may not be taken. Radiotherapy is usually offered as a follow-up treatment to this surgery, as is chemotherapy.

Mastectomy

If you have a modified radical mastectomy, all breast tissue is removed, including skin and lymph nodes. The muscles which support the breast are left intact. A simple mastectomy removes the breast tissue but may leave the skin, nipple and/or nodes and can be used in some cases of *in situ* diagnosis. This procedure is also known as a total mastectomy or a subcutaneous mastectomy. A total glandular mastectomy removes all the breast tissue, leaving the skin – but the nipple may be either removed or cored and replaced, leaving the areola (the darker skin that surrounds the nipple). Lymph nodes may or may not be taken. You may not need to have radiotherapy with this surgery but chemotherapy is generally offered, except in cases of DCIS.

Axillary clearance

Also known as axillary node dissection or lymph node removal. Depending on the pathology report, some or all of the underarm lymph nodes will be removed and analysed to determine the amount, if any, of lymph node involvement. This can be an indication of how much, if at all, the cancer has spread to secondary sites within the body and will be a factor in deciding the overall course of treatment following surgery.

After surgery

As many nerve-endings are severed during a mastectomy, many women are surprised at how little pain they feel following the surgery. The most inconvenient part of the surgery is dealing with the tubes and drains that remain in place for a few days after you leave hospital. The nurses empty the drains during your stay in hospital but it is up to you to do it when you leave. The drains are removed by your nurse or doctor at your first or second post-op check-up.

The first time you look at your surgery incision can be very daunting. Some women do so immediately the bandages are removed or changed and are very happy with the result, for others it is a longer process. If you have immediate reconstruction, the feeling of 'loss' is not so obvious and this option is highly recommended.

As the body, and therefore the skin, has an amazing ability to heal, you will be surprised at how normal your scar tissue will look in a matter of weeks or even days.

Following surgery, while you are in hospital and indeed when it is time for you to leave, you will be given some physio exercises. The standard exercise after a mastectomy is walking your fingers up a wall, increasing the height you reach each time. At first, you may find you feel very stiff on the side you have had surgery, but each day you will see a progression. It is important to carry on with these exercises when you leave hospital and try to use your arm as normally as possible once you have been checked by the doctor. Your mastectomy shouldn't limit the type of activity you do – professional athletes have been known to be back in training within six weeks.

You may also be given a temporary prosthesis on leaving the hospital, if you have not had immediate reconstruction. Normally, they are soft, lightweight, tear-drop-shaped and filled with fibre. Shoulder pads have been known to be substituted at times, especially when used with a mastectomy bra (a bra with an extra pocket for the prosthesis). After a few months, when the post-operative swelling has subsided, you can be fitted for a more permanent prosthesis and there are many varieties, shapes and sizes, including one for swimming.

Staging

Once a biopsy has been carried out and further surgery performed, the cancer can be staged according to its progression. Staging will depend on several factors, including whether the tumour is *in situ* or invasive, the number of nodes involved, the size of the tumour and whether there is any indication of spread to secondary sites throughout the body. Staging is necessary in order to determine the best adjuvant (follow-up) treatment.

Stage 0: DCIS

Stage I: A grape-sized tumour (about 2cm) that has not spread outside the breast

Stage II: A tumour of less than 2cm that has spread to the lymph nodes *or* a tumour between 2cm and 5cm that may or may not have spread to the lymph nodes *or* a tumour greater than 5cm with no spread to the lymph nodes

Stage III: (A) Smaller than 5cm but with considerable spread to the lymph nodes; (B) Cancer that has spread to tissue near the breast and/or lymph nodes near the collar bone

Stage IV: Inflammatory breast cancer or tumour that has spread to other parts of the body, mostly the bones, lungs and liver

(Source: International Union Against Cancer and the American Joint Committee on Cancer; *The Breast Cancer Companion*, LaTour)

Adjuvant treatment

Adjuvant treatment is follow-up treatment when there is no evidence of disease (NED) following surgery.

Radiotherapy

Radiotherapy uses X-rays to kill any remaining cancer cells in the local area, following surgery. It is most often used in conjunction with a lumpectomy. Sometimes it is used after a mastectomy when a tumour is close to the chest wall, leaving a very small margin of normal tissue between the tumour and the wall. Treatment is usually offered in short daily bursts over a period of weeks.

Reaction to radiotherapy varies from woman to woman, but some common side-effects include fatigue, itching in the local area of treatment, hair loss in the treated area (armpits, for example), a sunburn-type reaction or reddening of the skin – all of which are manageable and treatable.

Chemotherapy

Chemotherapy is a systemic treatment using drugs that seek out and destroy microscopic cancer cells, to stop secondary tumours developing or to shrink existing large tumours. Drugs are introduced into the bloodstream via intravenous injection, catheters (also known as central lines) or shunts (ports). In most breast cancer cases, chemotherapy is usually given every three weeks for 6–8 courses and chemotherapy is now standard treatment for Stages I and II breast cancers.

As the drugs can cause hardening and scarring of veins, sometimes a catheter or shunt (which is placed under the skin near the collar bone) will be recommended to patients who will undergo prolonged periods of chemotherapy, or to patients who already have small veins. A catheter also introduces the drugs into the system more slowly, over a longer period of time, so may be beneficial to patients who have very adverse reactions to the chemotherapy.

There are hundreds of types of chemotherapy drugs, each used for a specific purpose, according to the type of cancer diagnosed, and all with differing side-effects. Each woman's reaction to chemotherapy varies widely and no one else's should be taken as an indication of how you will feel during your treatment. Nowadays, anti-sickness medication stops most chemotherapy-induced nausea and vomiting, and an ice-cap (a frozen filled inflatable cap that is worn during chemotherapy sessions) can protect against complete hair loss.

There are many wigs available for women who do suffer from complete hair loss. Use this time to experiment and try a different style or colour for fun – it won't be so easy to do with your own hair! Many women prefer to go 'au naturel' or use a combination of hats, caps and scarves. As soon as your chemotherapy stops, your hair starts to grow immediately.

Fatigue and infection are the other side-effects that can be experienced during treatment. Making sure you get plenty of rest and help with daily chores during chemotherapy can help subdue feelings of tiredness. Susceptibility to infection can be a side-effect of treatment, caused when white blood cell counts hit their lowest point, about 14 days after the chemotherapy is given. As the white blood cells are responsible for fighting infection, when they are at their lowest your body is inhibited in its fight against any infection you are exposed to. During this cycle of your treatment, avoid overcrowded public areas, or people who are known to be infectious, and consult with your doctor at the first sign of fever or infection.

Hormone therapy

Hormone therapy is being hailed as the latest miracle cancer treatment, especially the oestrogen-blocking tamoxifen. Such drugs reduce the hormones that affect the growth of cancer cells in breast cancer. They are usually taken in tablet form.

There are some side-effects to these drugs but many would argue, as with chemotherapy, that the benefits of long-term survival far outweigh the downside. Side-effects of tamoxifen can include menopausal symptoms, such as irregular periods or lack of menstruation, hot flushes, vaginal dryness, mood swings and, very rarely, an increase in the incidence of endometrial cancer. Hormone replacement therapy (HRT) is now considered an option for women with breast cancer, and will alleviate many of these symptoms.

Bone marrow transplant

Bone marrow transplant is used with high-dose chemotherapy in high-risk patients (those with a high risk of recurrence). High-dose chemotherapy would wipe out the patient's own bone marrow, leaving them susceptible to critical infections, so it is removed from the patient ('harvested') before the chemotherapy is given. The bone marrow is then reintroduced after the chemotherapy has finished. Long periods in hospital are required, as well as periods in isolation units, to protect against contracting other infections.

Reconstruction

Nowadays, most women are offered the chance to have reconstruction either at the same time as their mastectomies (or lumpectomies), if they are suitable candidates, or a little while afterwards. It is a personal decision for you to contemplate, but most women who have had reconstruction are amazed and very happy with their cosmetic results.

Breast reconstruction should only be performed by experienced and qualified plastic surgeons who are highly recommended, and should only be carried out in consultation with your breast cancer surgeon. Many cancer hospitals work closely with a specialist breast plastic surgeon and, where available, their expertise should be sought.

As there are many methods of reconstruction, with varying degrees of surgery and recovery time, you should give great consideration to the type of reconstruction you want to have. The following is a guideline to these different forms of reconstruction.

Expander reconstruction

This is used following a modified radical mastectomy where skin has been removed as well as the breast tissue. An expander is a saline implant that is placed beneath the remaining skin and chest muscle. Saline solution is slowly injected into the implant over a period of weeks to gently stretch the remaining skin, to match the other breast. When the correct size is reached, the expander is removed and a permanent breast implant is inserted in its place.

Implant reconstruction

When enough skin has been saved during a mastectomy, an implant (either saline or silicone or both) is inserted under the skin and chest muscle.

Latissimus flap (back flap) reconstruction

The *Latissimus dorsi* (back muscle) is moved, with its skin, to the site of the breast and sewn into place, leaving the original blood supply intact. The eye-shaped tissue can be augmented with an implant beneath it.

Transverse *Rectus abdominis* myocutaneous flap reconstruction (TRAM)

Skin, muscle and fat are taken from the abdominal area, keeping the same blood supply, and tunnelled up to the breast area under the skin.

Nipple reconstruction

Skin from the groin area or behind the earlobe is attached to the breast mound to form a nipple and areola and then tattooed, to match the colour of the other nipple. Alternatively, existing skin can be pinched to form the nipple and the surrounding area tattooed to form the areola.

Breast implants

The safety of silicone breast implants has been a topic of controversy for many years, especially in the media. Many silicone implant manufacturers in the US have had to remove their products from the market owing to expensive litigation. In the UK, silicone implants are more freely available but in the US they are only available for use in breast reconstruction following cancer.

There is no conclusive evidence to suggest that silicone causes harm. Many plastic surgeons and breast cancer specialists who see women with silicone or silicone/saline implants every day report no incidence of illness caused by the implants. It appears to be an extremely small minority of women who have experienced problems.

It is a sad fact that the women who maintain that silicone implants are deadly and life-threatening are women who have had implants not for breast reconstruction following cancer but for personal vanity. Indeed, most of the women who campaign to have silicone implants removed from the market have not experienced the loss of their breasts and have no idea of the consequences for women with breast cancer of banning the implants.

On a more positive note, there are some excellent implants that combine silicone gel and saline to produce a natural-looking breast. These implants have a saline barrier surrounding the silicone gel, thus reducing any risk of silicone leakage.

Resources (for details see Recommended Books)
The Breast Cancer Companion (LaTour)
Cancer of the Breast (Royal Marsden)

COMPLEMENTARY THERAPIES

Many of the contributors to this book took some control back into their lives by seeking ways to strengthen their bodies to cope with the onslaught of surgery and treatment. Many looked towards complementary therapies.

Complementary therapies can help boost the immune system, making the body fight back naturally. When the immune system is strong it can assist in fighting the cancer cells.

As stress is a big inhibitor of the immune system, many complementary therapies aid relaxation. Good nutrition is also important in building up the system, helping build special blood cells that are effective in fighting cancer.

While some of these therapies could also be considered alternative – that is, they have been used in place of conventional cancer medical treatments – we recommend that they form complementary treatments, in addition to your orthodox medicine, with your doctor's approval.

Here are some of the more popular therapies.

Acupuncture

This is a 5,000-year-old Chinese tradition that unblocks stagnant energy in the body, in the organs and channels, promoting a healthy flow of energy, known as Qi.

Qi (or chi, pronounced 'chee') is the vital energy within the body as well as in all living organisms and it is the source of all movement and change.

Acupuncture uses very fine needles which are inserted into the skin to release this blocked energy.

Aromatherapy

The origin of aromatherapy dates back 5,000 years to ancient Egypt and India where essential oils were used for healing, in cosmetics and perfumes and for religious rites. Aromatherapy helps with emotional disorders by reducing stress, enhancing relaxation and relieving anxiety.

Chinese herbs

Chinese herbs make use of natural plant materials in the treatment of several ailments. The herbs can be taken raw, or steeped to make a tea, or taken in pill or capsule form.

There are many herbs and many uses, but some are of particular benefit in treating the unwanted effects of chemotherapy and radiotherapy, again with your doctor's approval.

- Ginseng and astragalus (Huang Qi) have anti-tumour properties and enhance the immune system by supporting the spleen and stomach.

- Shitake, reishi and maitake mushrooms also have anti-tumour properties and help strengthen and repair the immune system.

- Dandelion, used as greens, a tea or wine, helps improve Qi and aids in the detoxification of the body.

- Echinacea stimulates the immune system and is used as an antibiotic against infection.

- Green tea stimulates antioxidants and detoxifies enzymes.

Herbalism

Similar to Chinese herbs, Western herbalism uses plant extracts, vitamins and minerals for prevention and cure of illness. It works on the principle of fixing the problem, not just alleviating the symptoms.

- St John's Wort oil helps to keep the skin soft and supple, when used after radiotherapy.

- Milk thistle repairs damage to the liver caused by chemotherapy.

Homeopathy

Founded in the late eighteenth century by German physician Samuel

Hahnemann, homeopathy is based on the principle, similar to that behind vaccinations, of like curing like. Diluted substances that are given to patients suffering from certain ailments are found to cure them, although if given to a healthy person would make them suffer the same symptoms. Homeopathy teaches the body to learn to heal itself by stimulating the body's natural defence.

Qigong

This therapy uses a group of exercises to cultivate energy, improving health and longevity. It involves four principles, using mind and eye for meditation, movement in the form of gymnastics and breath in breath control. It helps restore harmony within our bodies and also with nature.

Yoga

This is another therapy practised for over 5,000 years. Like Qigong, it opens the medians in the body to keep the Qi (energy) flowing, releasing stagnant energy, increasing longevity and preventing disease.

There are many other therapies that are helpful in the treatment of breast cancer and they can be found on two very good websites:

- Swallows – complementary therapies for breast cancer – can be found at www.bcsupport.freeserve.co.uk

- Information about complementary and alternative medicine can be found at www.healingpeople.com

Resources (for details see Recommended Books)
Alternative Medicine: The Definitive Guide to Cancer (Diamond et al.)
Everybody's Guide to Homeopathic Medicine (Cummings and Ullman)
Healing and the Mind (Moyers)
Homeopathic Medicine at Home (Panos and Heimlich)

DIET AND NUTRITION

Guide to healthy eating

Eat more plant-based foods. They should make up 50 per cent of each of your meals. Try eating five servings of fresh fruit and vegetables per day, especially the yellow, green and red varieties.

Vegetables and pulses should include:

asparagus	cabbage	onions
aubergine	carrots	peas
beans	cauliflower	peppers
beetroot	courgettes	pumpkin
bok choy	cress	spinach
broccoli	garlic	sweet potatoes
Brussels sprouts	green beans	turnips
butternut squash	lentils	

Fruits should include:

apples	grapes	pineapple
bananas	kiwi	plums
blueberries	mango	prunes
cantaloupe	nectarines	raisins
cherries	oranges	raspberries
figs	peaches	strawberries
grapefruit	pears	tomatoes

Reduce your intake of red meat and **eat more** fish and lean meat. These should make up 25 per cent of your meal. Include:

bluefish	shellfish	chicken (remove
cod	striped bass	skin)
mackerel	trout	turkey
salmon	tuna	lean pork

Eat more grains and fibre. They should make up 25 per cent of your meal. Include:

rice
beans
wholegrain breads and cereals
oatmeal
pasta

Limit fat, sugar, salt, sweets and desserts.

Avoid bacon, sausage, ribs, crisps, cheese, cream, ice cream.

Avoid seed oils (corn, soybean, sunflower, safflower, cottonseed). **Use** canola oil, flaxseed oil, olive oil and walnut oil for cooking and spreading.

Avoid dairy products. **Use** skimmed milk, low-fat yoghurts, soymilk.

Drink 8–10 glasses of fluids each day. Include:

water (spring, mineral, seltzer)
fruit juice (apple, apricot, guava, grapefruit, orange, papaya, peach)
milk (skimmed)
vegetable juice
decaffeinated coffee
black and green tea

Avoid alcohol.

Macrobiotic diet

The macrobiotic diet is similar to a healthy-eating diet with an increase in fibre, fruit and vegetables and a reduction in the amount of fat, protein, salt and sugar. Macrobiotics aims to balance the elements of yin and yang in the diet, thereby balancing the energy in the body. Yin foods tend to be lighter, sweet foods such as fruit and vegetables; yang foods are heavier such as meat and dairy products.

The diet consists of:

- 50 per cent whole cereal grains: brown rice, barley, millet, oats, corn, rye, wheat and buckwheat including small portions of pasta and noodles

- 20 per cent organic vegetables, which should mostly be cooked

- 5–10 per cent beans and sea vegetables: adzuki, chickpeas, lentils, kelp and seaweeds

- 5–10 per cent soups made from the vegetables, grains, beans

- miso, tamari, soy sauce and sea salt as seasonings

Gerson therapy diet

The Gerson therapy diet has been used in the treatment and cure of chronic illnesses by utilizing the body's own healing mechanism. Organic fruits and vegetables are made into thirteen fresh, raw juices daily (one per hour for thirteen hours) that provide the body with immediate nutrients. The theory behind this diet is that it promotes an intense detoxification. Wastes are eliminated in order to regenerate the liver, and the immune system is reactivated, restoring the body's natural defences with enzymes, minerals and hormones. Also a part of this diet are coffee or camomile enemas which again help with detoxifying the body.

Supplements

Some of the following supplements are thought to help repair the body following chemotherapy:

- Alkyrol (shark's liver oil): contains omega 3 essential fatty acids (EFAs), vitamins A, D, E and helps boost the immune system

- Astragalus (Huang Qi): stimulates the immune system and restores T-cells (infection-fighting cells in the blood) to normal

- CO Q10 (coenzyme Q10): creates the fuel that energizes the body by improving the use of oxygen uptake by the heart-muscle cells

- Echinacea: stimulates immune system to fight infection

- Milk thistle: repairs damaged liver

- N-Acetyl L-Cysteine: detoxifies the liver

- Soy: has anti-tumour properties

Resources (for details see Recommended Books)
Healing Foods (Daniel)
Nutrition and Health (Strang)
The Tao of Nutrition (Ni)
Book of Jook: Chinese Medical Porridges (Flaws)

BREAST CANCER AND PREGNANCY

Diagnosis during pregnancy

As many more women of childbearing age are diagnosed with breast cancer each year, it is inevitable that more diagnoses will take place when a women is pregnant and that young women who have experienced breast cancer will want to go on to conceive. These are new and different dilemmas for the patient and cancer specialists.

It used to be thought that a woman diagnosed with breast cancer while pregnant had a poor prognosis. However, this is not the case. What is an important indicator of survival is the stage of cancer when the diagnosis takes place.

In pregnancy, it is often harder to diagnose cancer, as there are so many other changes taking place in the breast. This can lead to a delayed diagnosis which can therefore have an adverse effect on the prognosis.

Other emotional issues have to be dealt with by a pregnant breast cancer patient, such as termination of the pregnancy. If the staging of the cancer dictates that necessary life-saving treatment is required immediately, it may be to the disadvantage of the developing foetus. In some situations both mastectomy and chemotherapy may be performed safely during pregnancy without any immediate harm to the foetus, although the long-term risks of chemotherapy during pregnancy are unknown. The radiotherapy that is offered with a lumpectomy is known to be harmful to the foetus.

Pregnancy after diagnosis

It is generally considered that pregnancy will not bring on a recurrence of breast cancer. However, in some cases, pregnancy following a diagnosis of breast cancer is not recommended.

The prognosis for women with Stages I and II cancers remains unchanged by a pregnancy. As most recurrences take place during the first two years following diagnosis, it is advisable to wait a few years before conceiving. Pregnancy is not advised for the Stage I or II patient only if she has a recurrence.

Should women with Stage III cancers wish to conceive, they should wait at least five years following diagnosis. Women with Stage IV cancers should not plan a future pregnancy and women who were diagnosed with positive lymph nodes are also discouraged from future pregnancies.

The fear of pregnancy is not to do with stimulation of the existing cancer but with the probability of a recurrence in the future of that particular type of cancer, demanding ongoing treatment and, perhaps, entailing a poor prognosis. This has to be taken into account for anyone considering pregnancy, no matter what stage of cancer she has had. The dilemma is not how the pregnancy will affect the cancer but whether the mother will survive long enough to see her child grow to adulthood.

That being said, having cancer dictates many lifestyle and quality-of-life changes – some of which have been described in this book – that can help in the maintenance of the disease. It follows, then, that if a woman's quality of life can be increased significantly by her having a baby, this can also increase the probability of a better long-term prognosis.

Resources (for details see Recommended Books)
'How subsequent pregnancy affects outcome in women with a prior breast cancer' (Danforth)

BREAST CANCER AND SEXUALITY

So many changes take place when a woman experiences breast cancer and so many emotions come into play that it can have a profound effect on a woman's sexual feelings.

First, there is the altered body image due to the effects of the surgery – both with a mastectomy and with a lumpectomy. Second, there are quite extreme hormonal changes, due to the effects of the chemotherapy and tamoxifen, similar to those caused by menopause. This can result in a lack of libido, vaginal dryness and thinning of the vaginal membranes – all of which can make sexual intercourse quite painful. Add to this the emotional rollercoaster of a diagnosis; the realization of mortality; the treatment – sometimes debilitating; the recovery period; and even the lack of sensation in the treated breasts. All these factors can have an adverse effect on a woman's sex drive.

Equally, it is often difficult for a woman's partner to know when or how to approach her following treatment. Many partners do not want to hurt their wives or girlfriends by making advances immediately following surgery, so they choose avoidance. The woman perceives this as rejection and loss of attraction, due to her altered body shape. This creates a vicious cycle where the woman loses self-esteem and confidence, further exacerbating the feelings of inadequacy and lack of sex drive which push her partner further away.

The good news is that some of these side-effects can be treated. HRT (hormone replacement therapy – see page 184) is now considered (although controversially) an option for some breast cancer patients and this can help to erase some of the problems mentioned, such as loss of libido and dryness.

Within a healthy, committed relationship, a woman can overcome her sexual reticence with the help of her partner. Loss of sensation in the breasts can be offset by experimenting to find other erogenous zones. We tend to focus on the breast and nipple for sexual stimulation but there are many other areas of the body that bring great pleasure.

Reconstruction is so advanced these days that, except for the scars (which fade with time), a reconstructed nipple and breast can look and feel far superior to the real thing. Reconstruction can help many women rebuild their body image and free them from low self-esteem and lack of confidence.

It can take time for a woman to rebuild the same intimacy she shared with her partner before the surgery and treatment, but one thing is for sure: 'It sorts out the men from the boys.'

Sex and the single girl is another area of great concern, especially with more and more younger women being diagnosed. It is difficult to know when is the right time for intimacy or, indeed, when to disclose that you have had breast cancer and bear the visible scars. Gone are the days of women hiding themselves away in a life of celibacy.

Fortunately, the women in this book have the paramount attitude, 'Have war wound will travel.' Nothing will hold them back from getting out there and enjoying life to the full. Some are in long-term relationships and others are embarking on new and unexplored territory. There are men out there who are sensitive to a woman's needs.

Sometimes, it takes the crisis of breast cancer to highlight to the single girl which men are the ones worth pursuing. Perhaps in the past they have sought out destructive relationships, whereas now, they realize life is precious and they haven't got time for time-wasters. They now seek out the men who they know are mature enough to join them on their adventures.

BREAST CANCER AND HORMONE REPLACEMENT THERAPY (HRT)

When a woman's ovaries stop working at around the age of 45–55 (when she has her last period) the level of the hormone oestrogen in her body drops. This is known as the menopause and can be accompanied by a multitude of symptoms including hot flushes, dizziness, palpitations, insomnia, nausea, headaches, night sweats, breathlessness, vaginal dryness, pain during intercourse and loss of libido. Long-term effects of menopause include osteoporosis (brittle bones) and an increased risk of heart disease.

These symptoms and effects can be very distressing whether experienced naturally (because of the woman's age) or artificially (because she has undergone chemotherapy and hormone treatment). HRT replaces the natural hormones of oestrogen and progestogen in the body and can therefore alleviate some of the distressing effects of menopause.

As research suggests that oestrogen may be involved in the growth of breast cancers, HRT for breast cancer patients is very controversial. There have as yet been no clinical trials carried out on women with breast cancer who take HRT, so the long-term risks and benefits are still unknown. Each case should be discussed on an individual basis with your cancer specialist.

The primary indications for use of HRT with breast cancer patients depends on the type of breast cancer as well as how severe the menopausal symptoms are – weighing the potential benefits against the potential risks.

Tamoxifen, used in the treatment of breast cancer, may cause some of the menopausal symptoms mentioned above because it inhibits the amount of oestrogen in the body, but it does give some protection against osteoporosis and heart disease.

Resources (for details see Recommended Books)
Hormone Replacement Therapy (Royal Marsden)
Breast Cancer Hormones and HRT (Mount Vernon)

LYMPHOEDEMA

When the lymph vessels become blocked by scar tissue from surgery or radiotherapy, or lymph nodes are removed, lymph (fluid) collects in the surrounding tissue causing swelling. This swelling in the tissues is called lymphoedema. Most often it affects the limbs and sometimes the trunk. Not everyone develops lymphoedema, but if a woman has had axillary lymph nodes removed during surgery for breast cancer, she would be wise to avoid lymphoedema by guarding against infection.

Lymphoedema is treated by taking care of your skin, washing daily and using a moisturizer to keep the skin supple. Moderate exercise and use of the limb can help increase the flow of lymph, preventing build-up. Compression hosiery or multilayered bandaging also prevents the build-up of lymph by providing an even pressure to the limb, which encourages muscles to pump the lymph away more effectively. Massage, either self-massage or manual lymph drainage performed by a specialist, helps stimulate the lymphatic system to find alternative routes to drain lymph away from the area.

On the side of your body where you've had breast cancer surgery you should avoid:

- injections or infusions;

- having blood taken;

- having blood pressure taken;

- cuts and grazes;

- insect bites and stings;

- scratches or bites from pets;

- non-essential operations;

- acupuncture;

- very hot or very cold baths and showers;

- burns, including sunburn;

- direct contact with ice and snow;

- tight clothing and jewellery.

If an infection does occur you may need to take a course of antibiotics.

Resources (for details see Recommended Books)
Lymphoedema (Royal Marsden)

GLOSSARY

adjuvant treatment/chemotherapy: given as a preventative measure following surgery and radiotherapy, when there is no evidence of disease left in the body; used to kill off any microscopic cancer cells that remain undetected

anti-emetic: a medicine used to help control vomiting

aspiration: using a needle or syringe to take a sample of cells

axillary clearance or dissection: the removal of lymph nodes from the axilla region (armpit)

benign tumour: a non-cancerous growth

biopsy: a medical procedure whereby tissue is removed to be examined under a microscope

blood count: a blood test that calculates the number of white and red blood cells and platelets in the body

bone marrow: tissue inside bones that manufactures white and red blood cells

cancer: a disease characterized by abnormal cell growth such as a malignant tumour

catheter: a plastic tube inserted into the body for injecting fluids such as chemotherapy drugs or for removing bodily fluids

chemotherapy: chemical therapy in the treatment of cancer to stop its growth or spread

clinical trials: controlled scientific studies using patients to compare experimental cancer treatments with conventional methods

compression hosiery: elastic sleeve or stocking used in the treatment of lymphoedema

CT or CAT scan: computed axial tomography scan which is an X-ray showing cross sections of the body

cryopreservation: freezing tissue for preservation and possible medical use in the future

cytology: examination of cells under a microscope

diagnosis: a procedure whereby the doctor determines the type of disease prior to treating it

essential fatty acids (EFAs): fatty acids which are not made by the body but are essential for it

fibroadenoma: an overgrowth of fibrous tissue

hormone replacement therapy (HRT): the use of the hormones oestrogen and progestogen to replace the natural hormones produced by a woman's body which are lost during menopause; used in the treatment of menopausal symptoms

hormones: substances released by one organ in the body that affect the function of other organs

hormonal therapy: the use of hormones in the treatment of cancer, to block the effect of other hormones in order to slow down the growth of the cancer

hospice: a home for terminally ill patients where they receive care in the last few days of life

immune system: the body's natural defence against germs and diseases

infusion: the slow delivery of chemotherapy drugs intravenously

intravenous: through a vein

Latissimus dorsi: large back muscle

lesion: a mass of cells

localized: (a cancer) remaining in its original site, with no evidence of spread elsewhere in the body

lumpectomy: removal of a breast lump and an area of normal tissue around it

lymphatic system: system of nodes and vessels that carry white blood cells, in the lymph fluid, around the body to fight infection

lymphoedema: swelling in tissues below the skin when lymph cannot drain away

malignant tumour: a cancerous growth

mammogram: an X-ray of breast tissue

manual lymph massage: massage that stimulates the lymphatic system to treat lymphoedema

mastectomy: removal of all breast tissue

metastasis: the spread of cancer from its original location to another site within the body

oncologist: a doctor who specializes in the treatment of cancer

palliative care: treatment given to help with pain associated with cancer rather than treating the cancer itself

primary tumour: the primary site of the cancer, which names it, e.g., breast cancer, regardless of whether it has spread elsewhere in the body

prognosis: the medical prediction of how well the patient will do in the future, based on statistics and the doctor's evaluation of the patient's condition

prosthesis: an artificial breast form

radiotherapy: the treatment of cancer using high-energy X-rays

Rectus abdominis: a muscle in the abdomen that runs from the breast bone to the pubic bone

recurrence: the reappearance of cancer after a period of remission

regression: the shrinkage of a tumour or the slowing down of its growth

staging: the evaluation of the cancer to determine its progression and possible spread throughout the body

systemic: (treatment) affecting the whole body

tamoxifen: hormone drug used to block oestrogen in the body to slow down or stop the growth of cancer

tumour: an abnormal mass of tissue that may be benign or malignant

tumour markers: blood tests that can indicate the status of a tumour

ultrasound scan: a scan that uses sound waves to build up a picture of the body

X-ray: electromagnetic radiation that passes through the body to provide an image of the inside and outside of the body

RECOMMENDED BOOKS

These books have been read and recommended by the contributors to this book.

The Alchemist, Paolo Coelho (Thorsons, 1995)

Alternative Medicine: The Definitive Guide to Cancer, W. John Diamond, W. Lee Cowden with Burton Goldberg (Future Medicine Publishing, 1997)

The Art of Happiness, The Dalai Lama and Howard Cutler (Coronet, 1999)

Book of Jook: Chinese Medical Porridges, Bob Flaws (Blue Poppy Press)

Breakthrough into Verse: A Book of Poems, Jenny Whiteside (Jenny Whiteside, 1997)

Breast Awareness, Breakthrough Breast Cancer (see Cancer Support Addresses)

The Breast Cancer Companion. From Diagnosis Through Treatment and Recovery: Everything You Need to Know for Every Step Along the Way, Kathy LaTour (Avon Books, NYC, USA, 1993)

Breast Cancer Hormones and HRT, Cancer Support Information, Mount Vernon Hospital (see Cancer Support Addresses)

Cancer of the Breast, Patient Information Series, Royal Marsden NHS Trust, London and Surrey (see Cancer Support Addresses)

The Chemotherapy Survival Guide, Judith McKay and Nancee Hirano (New Harbinger Publications Inc., CA, USA,1998)

The Creation of Health: The Emotional, Psychological and Spiritual Responses That Promote Health and Healing, Caroline Myss, Ph.D., and C. Norman Shealy, MD (Three Rivers Press, NYC, USA, 1993)

The Diary of Virginia Woolf, Anne Olivia Bell (ed.), Hogarth Press, 1995

Dr Susan Love's Breast Book, Susan M. Love et al. (Addison Wesley)

Eight Weeks to Optimum Health: A Proven Program for Taking Full Advantage of Your Body's Natural Healing Power, Andrew Weil, MD (Fawcett Columbine, NYC, USA, 1997)

Everybody's Guide to Homeopathic Medicine, Stephen Cummings and Dana Ullman

Everything You Need to Know About Breast Awareness, Patient Information Series, Royal Marsden NHS Trust, London and Surrey (see Cancer Support Addresses)

The Gold Cell, Sharon Olds (Alfred A. Knopf, 1987)

Guarding the Three Treasures: The Chinese Way of Health, Daniel Reid (Simon & Schuster, 1993)

A Guide for the Advanced Soul: A Book of Affirmations, Susan Hayward (In Tune Books, 1999)

'Harry Potter' series, J. K. Rowling (Bloomsbury, 1997, 1998, 1999, 2000)

Healing and the Mind, Bill Moyers (Doubleday, 1993)

Healing Foods: How to Nurture Yourself and Fight Illness, Dr Rosy Daniel (Thorsons, 1996)

Hiaasen, Carl, any book by, e.g., *Lucky You*; *Stormy Weather*; *Double Whammy*; *Strip Tease*; *Skin Tight*; *Kiss Ass: Selected Columns* (Picador/Pan) or *A Carl Hiaasen Collection* (Random House Audio, 2000)

Homeopathic Medicine at Home, Moesimund Panos and Jane Heimlich

Hormone Replacement Therapy, Patient Information Series, Royal Marsden NHS Trust, London and Surrey (see Cancer Support Addresses)

'How subsequent pregnancy affects outcome in women with a prior breast cancer', David N. Danforth, Jr., MD (*Oncology*, November 1991)

Jonathan Livingston Seagull, A Story, Richard Bach (HarperCollins, 1994)

Laughter Is the Best Therapy: Happiness Now, Robert Holden (Coronet, 1999)

Living Beyond Breast Cancer: A Survivor's Guide, Marisa C. Weis, MD, and Ellen Weis (Random House/Time Books)

Living With Cancer, Dr Rosy Daniel (Robinson, London, 2000)

Love, Medicine and Miracles, Bernie S. Siegel, MD (Arrow Books, London, 1986)

Lymphoedema, Patient Information Series, Royal Marsden NHS Trust, London and Surrey (see Cancer Support Addresses)

Making the Chemotherapy Decision, David Drum (Lowell House, CA, USA, 1996)

'The median isn't the message', Stephen Jay Gould in *Adam's Navel* (Penguin, 1995)

Nutrition and Health, Strang Cancer Prevention Center, NY (see Cancer Support Addresses)

Original Blessing, Matthew Fox

Prescriptions for Living, Bernie S. Siegel, MD (HarperCollins, 2000)

The Small Woman, Alan Burgess

Spontaneous Healing: How to Discover and Enhance Your Body's Natural Ability to Maintain and Heal Itself, Andrew Weil, MD (Fawcett Columbine, NYC, USA, 1995)

Springs of Hope: Book of Sayings (Herder and Herder, NY)

The Stone Diaries, Carol Shields (Fourth Estate, 1994)

The Tao of Nutrition, Dr Ni (Seven Star Communications)

The Way, Blessed Josemaria Escriva (Sceptre)

A Woman's Decision, Karen Berger and John Bostock III, MD (Quality Medical Publishing Inc.)

Women of Silence: The Emotional Healing of Breast Cancer, Grace Gawler (Hill of Content, 1994)

You Can Heal Your Life, Louise Hay (Eden Grove Editions, 1998)

FURTHER READING

The following books have been published either in the US or in the UK. This is by no means an exhaustive list of breast cancer books and does not constitute a recommended reading list, purely an indication of some of the books available.

The Answer is Within you: Psychology, Women's Connections and Breast Cancer, Lauren K. Ayers (Crossroad Publishing)

Art. Rage. Us: Art and Writing by Women With Breast Cancer (Chronicle Books)

Ask the Doctor: Breast Cancer, Vincent E. Friedewald et al. (Ask the Doctor Series, Andrews McMeel Publishing)

Atlas of Breast Imaging, Danial B. Kopans (Lippincott, Williams & Wilkins)

Atlas of Mammography: New Early Signs in Breast Cancer, Parvis Gamagami (Iowa State University Press)

Be a Survivor: Your Guide to Breast Cancer Treatment, Vladimir Lange (Lange Productions)

Better Breast Health Naturally with Chinese Medicine, Honora Lee Wolfe and Bob Flaws (Blue Poppy Press)

Breakthrough: The Race to Find the Breast Cancer Gene, Kevin Davies and Michael White (John Wiley & Sons)

Breast Cancer, Elaine Landau (Franklin Watts)

Breast Cancer, Lucille Pederson and Janet M. Trigg (Bergin & Garvey)

Breast Cancer, Daniel F. Roses (W. B. Saunders Company)

Breast Cancer, S. Eva Singletary and Raphael E. Pollock (eds) (Springer-Verlag TELOS)

Breast Cancer: All You Need to Know to Take an Active Part in Your Treatment, Karen Gelmon et al. (Gordon Soules Book Publishers)

Breast Cancer and Me: One Woman's Story of Victory over a Deadly Disease, Lois Olmstead (Christian Publications)

Breast Cancer and You: Bettering the Odds: How to Join the Increasing Number of Women Who Survive, Whole and Well, Martha Grigg (Branden Publishing)

Breast Cancer? Breast Health! The Wise Woman Way, Christine Northrup, MD (Wise Woman Herbal Series, Ash Tree)

Breast Cancer: The Complete Guide, Yasher Hirshaut, MD, and Peter Pressman, MD (Bantam)

The Breast Cancer Handbook – Taking Control After You've Found a Lump, Joan Swirsky and Barbara Balaban (Power Publications)

Breast Cancer: A Husband's Story, Bruce Sokol and John Falkenberry (Crane Hill Publishers))

Breast Cancer Journal: A Century of Petals, Juliet Wittman (Fulcrum Publishing)

Breast Cancer? Let Me Check My Schedule!, Peggy McCarthy et al. (eds) (HarperCollins)

Breast Cancer: Molecular Genetics, Pathogenesis and Therapeutics (Contemporary Cancer Research), Anne M. Bowcock (ed.) (Humana Press)

Breast Cancer: Myths and Facts. What You Need to Know, S. Eva Singletary and Alice F. Judkins, RN (PRR Inc.)

Breast Cancer: A Patient Guide, Patricia J. Anderson (Health Services)

Breast Cancer: Poisons, Profits and Prevention, Liane Clorfene-Casten (LPC Group)

The Breast Cancer Prevention and Recovery Diet, Suzannah Olivier (Michael Joseph)

The Breast Cancer Prevention Diet: The Powerful Foods, Supplements and Drugs That Can Save Your Life, Bob Arnot (Little, Brown)

The Breast Cancer Prevention Program, Samuel Epstein et al. (Macmillan)

The Breast Cancer Survival Manual: A Step-by-Step Guide for the Woman with Newly Diagnosed Breast Cancer, John Link (Owl Publishing)

Breast Cancer Survivors' Club: A Nurse's Experience, Lillie Shockney (Windsor House Publishing)

Breast Care Options for the 1990s, Paul Kuehn (Newmark Publishing)

Breast Care: The Woman's Guide to Cancer Prevention and Optimal Breast Health Through Nutrition and Lifestyle, Kate Gilbert Udall (Woodland Publishing)

Breast Disease, Douglas J. Marchant (ed.) (W. B. Saunders Company)

Breast Health/What You Need to Know About Disease Prevention, Diagnosis, Treatment, and Guidelines for Healthy Breast Care, Charles B. Simone (Avery Publishing)

Breast Imaging, Daniel B. Kopans (Rittenhouse Book Distributors Inc.)

Breast Imaging Companion, Gilda Cardenosa (Lippincott, Williams & Wilkins)

Breast Self-Examination, Albert R. Milan (Workman Publishing)

C-Notes: My Journey Through Breast Cancer, Patsy Paxton (Commonwealth Publishing)

Can You Come Here Where I Am? The Poetry and Prose of Seven Breast Cancer Survivors, Rita Busch et al. (eds) (EMPR Inc.)

Cancer as a Turning Point, Lawrance LeShan, Ph.D. (Dutton)

Cancer As Initiation: Surviving the Fire: A Guide for Living With Cancer for Patient, Provider, Spouse, Family or Friend, Barbara Stone (Open Court Publishing)

The Cancer Conqueror, Greg Anderson (Word)

Cancer in Women, John J. Kavanagh (ed.) (Blackwell Science Inc.)

The Cancer Journals, Audre Lorde (Aunt Lute Books)

Cancer Sourcebook for Women: Basic Information About Specific Forms of Cancer That Affect Women, Featuring Facts About Breast Cancer, Cervical . . . , Alan R. Cook and Peter D. Dresser (eds) (Omnigraphics)

Chinese System of Food Cures, Henry Lu (Ward Lock)

Choices, Marion Morra, Eve Potts (Avon Books)

Color Atlas of Breast Diseases, Robert E. Mansel and J. Nigel Bundred (Mosby Inc.)

The Complete Book of Breast Care, Niels H. Lauersen and Eileen Stukane (Fawcett Crest)

The Complete Breast Book, June Engel (Key Porter Books)

Contemporary Issues in Breast Cancer, Karen Hassey Doe (Jones & Bartlett)

Coping: A Young Woman's Guide to Breast Cancer Prevention, Bettijane Eisenpreis (Rosen Publishing)

Coping with Breast Cancer, Heyderman and Eadie (Sheldon Press)

Coping with Breast Cancer, Robert H. Phillips and Paula Goldstein (Avery Publishing)

Coping with Chemotherapy, Nancy Bruning (Ballantine Health)

A Darker Ribbon: Breast Cancer, Women and Their Doctors in the Twentieth Century, Ellen Leopold (Beacon Press)

Desperate Hope: Experiencing God in the Midst of Breast Cancer, Barbara Milligan (Intervarsity Press)

Diagnosis and Management of Breast Disease, Richard E. Blackwell and James C. Grotting (eds) (Iowa State University Press)

Diseases of the Breast, Jay R. Harris et al. (eds) (Lippincott, Williams & Wilkins)

Dressed to Kill: The Link Between Breast Cancer and Bras, Sydney Ross Singer and Soma Grismaijer (Avery Publishing)

The Enemy Within: The High Cost of Living Near Nuclear Reactors: Breast Cancer, Aids, Low Birthweights, and other Radiation-Induced Immune Deficiencies, Jay M. Gould et al. (eds) (Four Walls Eight Windows)

Estrogen and Breast Cancer: A Warning to Women, Carol Ann Rinzler (Hunter House Publishers)

Estrogen Antiestrogen Action and Breast Cancer Therapy, V. Craig Jordan (ed.) (University of Wisconsin Press)

Examining Myself: One Woman's Story of Breast Cancer Treatment and Recovery, Musa Mayer (Faber & Faber)

The Feisty Woman's Breast Cancer Book, Elaine Ratner (Hunter House)

Fine Black Lines: Reflections on Facing Cancer, Fear and Loneliness, Lois Tschetter Hjelmstad (Mulberry Hill)

The First Year of the Rest of Your Life: Reflections for Survivors of Breast Cancer, Charla Hudson Honea (ed.) (Pilgrim Press)

Five Stages of Getting Well, Judy Edwards Allen (Lifetime Publishing)

Getting Well Again, Stephanie Matthews-Simonton and Carl Simonton (Bantam)

The Guide to Cosmetic Surgery, Josleen Wilson (Simon & Schuster)

Held, an Angel's Wing: A Survival Handbook for Women with Breast Cancer, Raeia J. Hinson and Michael H. Hinson (Vital Issues Press)

Her-2: The Making of Herceptin, a Revolutionary Treatment for Breast Cancer, Robert Bazell (Random House)

Hollis Sigler's Breast Cancer Journal, Hollis Sigler et al. (Hudson Hills Press)

Hope Is Contagious: The Breast Cancer Treatment Survival Handbook, Margit Esser Porter (ed.) (Simon & Schuster)

How I Conquered Cancer Naturally, Eydie Mae and Chris Loeffler (Avery Publishing)

How to Prevent Breast Cancer, Ross Pelton et al. (Simon & Schuster)

Ideologies of Breast Cancer, Laura K. Potts (ed.) (Macmillan)

Ideologies of Breast Cancer: Feminist Perspectives, Laura K. Potts (ed.) (St Martin's Press)

I'm Alive and the Doctor's Dead: Surviving Cancer with Your Sense of Humor and Your Sexuality Intact, Sue Buchanan (Zondervan Publishing)

In God's Hand: One Woman's Experience with Breast Cancer, Becky Lynn Wecksler and Michael Wecksler (Herald Press)

In Honor of Women: A Revolutionary Approach to Prevent Breast Cancer and Other Diseases, Stella Togo Crawley (Ballantine)

The Journey Beyond Breast Cancer: From the Personal to the Political: Taking an Active Role in Prevention, Diagnosis, and Your Own Healing, Virginia M. Soffa (Inner Traditions Intl Ltd)

Keep Your Breasts: Preventing Breast Cancer the Natural Way, Susan Moss, MD, and James R. Privetara (Resource Publications)

Life Before Death, Abby Frucht (Scribner)

Living in the Postmastectomy Body: Learning to Live in and Love Your Body Again, Rebecca Zuckweiler (Hartley & Marks Publishers)

Living on the Margins: Women Writers on Breast Cancer, Hilda Raz (ed.) (Persea Books Inc.)

Love, Judy: Letters of Hope and Healing for Women with Breast Cancer, Judy Hart (Conari Press)

A Matter of Heart: One Woman's Triumph Over Breast Cancer and a Heart Transplant, Nancy Shank Pedder (Saturn Press)

Medicine and Meaning, Larry Dossey, MD (Bantam)

Michael's Mommy Has Breast Cancer, Lisa Torrey and Barbara W. Watler (Hibiscus Press)

My Healing from Breast Cancer, Barbara Joseph (Keats Publishing)

My Mother's Breast: Daughters Face their Mother's Cancer, Laurie Tarkan (Taylor Publishing)

No Mountain Too High: A Triumph over Breast Cancer: The Story of the Women of Expedition Inspiration, Andrea Gabbard (Adventura Books, Seal Press)

The Not-So-Scary Breast Cancer Book: Two Sisters' Guide from Discovery to Recovery, Carolyn Ingram et al. (Impact Publishers)

Now Breathe: A Very Personal Journey Through Breast Cancer, Claudia Sternbach (Whiteaker Press)

Ordinary Life: A Memoir of Illness, Kathlyn Conway (W. H. Freeman & Company)

Pathology of the Breast, Fattaneh A. Tavassoli (Prentice Hall)

Patient No More: The Politics of Breast Cancer, Sharon Batt (Gynergy Books/Ragweed Press)

Pink Ribbon Quilts: A Book Because of Breast Cancer, Mimi Dietrich (Martingale & Company)

Preventing Breast Cancer, Cathy Read (Oram Press/Pandora)

Preventing Breast Cancer: The Story of a Major, Proven, Preventable Cause of This Disease, John W. Gofman and Egan O'Conner (eds) (Committee Nuclear Responsibility)

Quantum Healing, Deepak Chopra (Bantam)

The Race is Run One Step at a Time: Every Woman's Guide to Taking Charge of Breast Cancer and My Personal Story, Nancy G. Brinker and Catherine McEvilly Harris (Summit Publishing)

Rainbow of Hope, Marie Eckess (Winepress Publishing)

Reclaiming Our Lives After Breast and Gynecologic Cancer, Kristine Falco (Jason Aronson Inc.)

Recovering from Breast Surgery: Exercises to Strengthen Your Body and Relieve Pain, Diana Stumm (Hunter House)

Recovering the Soul, Larry Dossey, MD (Bantam)

The Red Devil: To Hell with Cancer – And Back, Katherine Russell Rich (Crown Publishers Inc.)

The Road Back to Health, Neil A. Fiore, Ph.D. (Bantam)

A Safe Place: A Journal for Women With Breast Cancer, Jennifer Pike (Chronicle Books)

She Came to Live Out Loud: An Inspiring Family Journey Through Illness, Loss and Grief, Myra MacPherson (Scribner)

Speak the Language of Healing: Living With Breast Cancer Without Going to War, Susan Kuner et al. (eds) (Conari Press)

Spinning Straw into Gold: Your Emotional Recovery from Breast Cancer, Ronnie Kaye (Simon & Schuster)

A Step-by-Step Guide to Dealing With Your Breast Cancer, Rebecca Y. Robinson and Jeanne A. Petrek (Citadel Press)

Straight from the Heart: Letters of Hope and Inspiration from Survivors of Breast Cancer, Ina L. Yalof (ed.) (Kensington Publishing)

Straight Talk About Breast Cancer: From Diagnosis to Recovery: A Guide for the Entire Family, Suzanne W. Braddock and John J. Edney (Addicus Books)

Survivor's Guide to Breast Cancer: A Couple's Story of Faith, Hope & Love, Robert C. Fore et al. (Peake Road)

Tamoxifen and Breast Cancer, Michael Degregorio and Valerie Wiebe (Yale)

Tamoxifen: New Hope in the Fight Against Breast Cancer, John F. Kessler and Greg A. Annussek (Avon Books)

This Adventure Called Life: Healing from Breast Cancer Naturally, Peny Goodson-Kjome and Ann Franco-Ferriera (illustrator) (SunShine Press Publications)

To Run the Race With Joy, Sandy Rice (CSS Publishing)

Total Breast Health: The Power Food Solution for Protection and Wellness, Robin Keuneke (Kensington Publishing)

Traditional Chinese Medicine: A Woman's Guide to Healing from Breast Cancer, Nan Lu and Ellen Schaplowsky (HarperCollins)

Tree: Essays and Pieces, Deena Metzger (North Atlantic Books)

Triumph, Getting Back to Normal When You Have Cancer, Marion Morra and Eve Potts (Avon Books)

The Truth About Breast Cancer, Hay and Claire Hoy (Stoddart)

The Truth About Breast Cancer: A Seven Step Prevention Plan, Joseph Keon (Parissound Publishing)

Ultimate Living!, Dee Simmons (Creation House Press Breast Cancer Support Directory)

Understanding Breast Cancer Risk, Patricia T. Kelly (Health, Society and Policy Series, Temple University Press)

The Unofficial Guide to Surviving Breast Cancer, Dr Richard Theriault (Macmillan)

Victory Through Breast Cancer, Glenda B. Sumerel (Sumerel Enterprises)

Woman to Woman: A Handbook for Women Newly Diagnosed With Breast Cancer, Hester Hill Schnipper, LICSW, and Joan Feinberg Berns (Avon Books)

Women Confront Cancer: Making Medical History, Choosing Alternative and Complementary, Margaret J. Wooddell and David J. Hess (eds) (New York University Press)

CANCER SUPPORT ADDRESSES

Action Cancer (clinic, screening, counselling)
1 Marlborough Park
Belfast BT9 6HQ
Tel: 01232 661081

Amarant Trust (menopause and HRT)
11–13 Charterhouse Buildings
London EC1M 7AN
Tel: 01293 413000
24-hour info: 0891 660620 (39p per min. cheap rate; 49p per min. at other times)

Amoena (nipples and prostheses)
Amoena (UK) Ltd
14–15 Monks Brook Park
Scholl Close
Chandlers Ford
Eastleigh
Hampshire SO53 4RA
Tel: 0170 327 0345/ 0800 378 668

Anita International Ltd (prostheses and swimwear)
15–16a Eton Garages
Eton Avenue
London NW3 4PE
Tel: 020 7435 2258

Aromatherapy Organizations Council
3 Latymer Close
Braybrokke
Market Harborough
Leicestershire LE16 8LN
Tel: 01858 434242

Bach Flower Centre
Mount Vernon
Baker's Lane
Brightwell-cum-Sotwell
Wallingford
Oxfordshire OX10 0PZ
Tel: 01491 834678
Mail Order: 020 7495 2404

Breakthrough Breast Cancer (charity funding research)
Kingsway House
103 Kingsway
London WC2B 6QX
Tel: 020 7405 5111
Fax: 020 7831 3873
website: www.breakthrough.org.uk

Breast Cancer Care (support charity)
Kiln House
210 New King's Road
London SW6 4NZ
Tel: 020 7384 2984
Freephone: 0500 245345
e-mail: information@breastcancer care.org.uk
website: www.breastcancercare. org.uk

also at: 46 Gordon Street
Glasgow G1 3PU
Tel: 0141 221 2233

Breast Cancer Coalition
PO BOX 8554
London SW8 2ZB
Tel: 020 7720 0945
Fax: 020 7720 8877

Breast Cancer Support Website
(excellent resource website)
www.bcsupport.freeserve.co.uk/
swallows.html

Bristol Cancer Help Centre (holistic
therapies)
Grove House
Cornwallis Grove
Clifton
Bristol BS8 4PG
Tel: 0117 980 9500
Helpline: 0117 980 9505
Shop: 0117 980 9504
Bookings: 0117 980 9050
Dr Rosy Daniel, consultations:
London 020 7299 9428
Bristol 0117 980 9521

British Association of Aesthetic
Surgeons (plastic surgeon
directory)
The Royal College of Surgeons
35 Lincoln's Inn Fields
London WC2A 3PA
Tel: 020 7831 5161

British Association of Art Therapists
01710 383 3774

British Association of Counsellors
01788 578328

British Council of Acupuncture
020 8735 0400

British Reflexology Association
01886 821207

British Wheel of Yoga
01529 306851

Cancer Alternative Information
Bureau (alternative therapies)
020 7266 1505

Cancer Research Campaign
Freephone: 0800 226 237
website: www.crc.org.uk

cancerBACUP (free counselling)
3 Bath Place
Rivington Street
London EC2A 3JR
Tel: 020 7613 2121
30 Bell Street
Glasgow G11LG
Tel: 0141 553 1553

Cancerlink (support groups)
11–21 Northdown Street
London N1 9BN
Tel: 020 7520 2603/020 7520 2606
Fax: 020 7833 4963
Freephone: 0800 132905
e-mail: Cancerlink@canlink.demon.
co.uk

Cancer Support Centre Wandsworth
(holistic support)
PO BOX 17
20–22 York Road
London SW11 3QE
Helpline: 020 7924 3924
Fax: 020 7978 6505

Carers' National Association
(support for carers)
20–25 Glasshouse Yard
London EC1A 4JS
Tel: 020 7490 8898
Information: 0345 573369

Christie Hospital, Manchester
website: www.christie.man.ac.uk

Cruse Bereavement Care
(counselling)
126 Sheen Road
Richmond
Surrey TW9 1UR
020 8940 4818
Helpline: 020 8332 7227

Disabled Living Foundation
380–384 Harrow Road
London W9 2HU
Tel: 020 7289 6111
Freephone: 0808 800 1234
website: www.cancerbacup.org.uk

Gray Laboratory, Mount Vernon
Hospital
website: www.graylab.ac.uk

Haven Trust (support)
020 7384 0000

Hospice Information Service at
St Christopher's
St Christopher's Hospice
51–59 Lawrie Park Road
Sydenham
London SE26 6DZ
020 8778 9252

Imperial Cancer Research
PO BOX 123
Lincoln's Inn Fields
London WC2A 3PX
Tel: 020 7242 0200
Tel: 020 7269 3611
website: www.icnet.uk/

Inamed Ltd (breast implant info)
Customer Services Department
Unit 4 Forest Court
Fishponds Estate
Fishponds Road
Wokingham
Berkshire RG41 2QJ
Tel: 0118 977 0022

Institute for Optimum Nutrition
Blades Court
Deodar Road
London SW15 2NU
Tel: 020 8877 9993

Institute of Cancer Research
Freephone: 0800 731 9468
website: www.icr.ac.uk/icrhome

Institute of Complementary
Medicine
PO BOX 194
London SE16
Tel: 020 7237 5165

Irish Cancer Society
5 Northumberland Road
Dublin
Tel: 00353 1668 1855
Fax: 00353 1668 7599
Helpline: 800 200 700

Lavender Trust (for young women
with breast cancer)
c/o Breast Cancer Care
Freepost LON 644
London SW6 4BR
Tel: 020 7384 2984
website: www.lavendertrustfund.
org.uk

Lymphoedema Support Network
St Luke's Crypt
Sydney Street
London SW3 6NH
Helpline: 0707 122 4760
Tel: 020 7351 4480
Fax: 020 7349 9809
website: www.lymphoedema.
  org.lsn

Macmillan Cancer Relief (provides
  specialist carers)
Anchor House
15/19 Britten Street
London
SW3 3TZ
Tel: 020 7351 7811
Fax: 020 7376 8098
e-mail: informationline@macmillan.
  org.uk
website: www.macmillan.org.uk
Information: 0845 601 6161

Marie Curie Cancer Care (provides
  nurses and hospices)
28 Belgrave Square
London EC2A 3AR
Tel: 020 7235 3325
Fax: 020 7823 2380/ 235 2297
website: www.mariecurie.org.uk

Mount Vernon Hospital
Rickmansworth Road
Northwood
Middlesex HA6 2RN
Tel: 01923 826111

National Cancer Alliance (provides
  cancer specialist directory)
PO BOX 579
Oxford OX4 1LB
Tel: 01865 793566

National Institute of Medical
  Herbalists
56 Longbrook Street
Exeter EX4 6AH
Tel: 01392 426022

National Osteoporosis Society
PO BOX 10
Radstock
Bath BA3 3YB
Helpline: 01761 472721

Neal's Yard Agency (advice on
  workshops, courses, counselling)
14 Neal's Yard
London WC2H 9DP
Tel: 07000 783704

Neal's Yard Remedies
15 Neal's Yard
London WC2H 9DP
Tel: 020 7379 7222
Mail order: 01865 245 436

Nearly Me Nipples
Medimac Ltd
15–16 St Mary's House
St Mary's Road
Shoreham by Sea
West Sussex BN43 5ZA
Tel: 01273 441436

Nicola Jane (bras and swimwear)
Forum House
Stirling Road
Chichester
West Sussex PO19 2EN

also at: Lagness
Chichester
West Sussex PO20 6LW
Tel: 01243 268686
Freephone: 0800 018 2121

Radiotherapy Action Group
Exposure
Tel: 020 8460 7476 (breast cancer)

Research Council for
Complementary Medicine
60 Great Ormond Street
London WC1N 3JF
Tel: 020 7833 8897

Rigby and Peller (specialist bra
makers)
2 Hans Road
London SW3 1RX
Tel: 020 7589 9293

Royal Free Hospital
website: www.vois.org.uk/
cancerkin

Royal London Homoeopathic
Hospital
Great Ormond Street
London WC1N 3HR
Tel: 020 7837 8833

Royal Marsden Hospital
website: www.royalmarsden.org/

Shiatsu Society
01733 758341

Society for the Promotion of
Nutritional Therapy
PO BOX 47
Heathfield
East Sussex TN21 8ZX
Tel: 01825 872921

Society of Homoeopaths
4A Artizan Road
Northampton
NN1 4HU
Tel: 01604 621400

Strang Cancer Prevention Center
428 East 72nd Street
New York
NY 10021
USA
Tel: 001 212 746 6629

Sue Ryder Foundation (provides
hospices)
Cavendish
Sudbury
Suffolk CO10 8AY
Tel: 01787 280252

Tak Tent Cancer Support Scotland
The Western Infirmary
Block C20 Western Court
100 University Place
Glasgow G12 6SQ
Tel: 0141 211 1932

Tamoxifen (the facts)
Tenovus
11 Whitechurch Road
Cardiff CF4 3JN
Freephone helpline: 0800 526527

Tenovus Cancer Information Centre
PO BOX 887
College Buildings
Courtenay Road
Cardiff CF1 1FA
Tel: 01222 497 7000
Fax: 01222 489919
Freephone helpline: 0800 526527

Trulife Ltd (prostheses and nipples)
4a Beechers Drive
Aintree Racecourse Business Park
Liverpool L9 5YA
Tel: 0151 525 9200

Ulster Cancer Foundation
40–42 Eglantine Avenue
Belfast BT9 6DX
Tel: 01232 660081
Helpline: 01232 663439

Women's Health
52–54 Featherstone Street
London EC1Y 8RT
Tel: 020 7251 6580

Women's Nationwide Cancer
Control Campaign (supports early
    diagnosis)
Suna House
128–130 Curtain Road
London EC2A 3AR
Tel: 020 7729 4688
Fax: 020 7613 0771
Helpline: 020 7729 2229

Women's Nutritional Advisory
    Service
Tel: 01273 487666

www.healingpeople.com
    (excellent US website for details
    of complementary medicine)

BREAKTHROUGH CHALLENGE

Breakthrough Breast Cancer is a charity committed to fighting breast cancer through research and awareness and has established the UK's first dedicated breast cancer research centre. The Breakthrough Toby Robins Breast Cancer Research Centre opened in December 1999 at the Institute of Cancer Research and is associated with the renowned Royal Marsden Hospital in London. This puts it at the very heart of the largest cancer complex in Europe.

Breakthrough also campaigns to keep breast cancer at the top of the public and political agendas, promoting education and awareness of the issue among the public, policy-makers, health professionals and the media.

Breakthrough has an innovative approach to fundraising. Our most high-profile and successful fundraising campaign is Fashion Targets Breast Cancer, which has raised more than £3 million. In addition, thousands of individual supporters and a network of groups across the country have raised millions of pounds through a wide range of fundraising initiatives, such as the £1,000 Challenge.

Despite Breakthrough's achievements over the past nine years, there is still a long way to go. The establishment of the Breakthrough Research Centre is the beginning of a long journey towards our ultimate goal – a future free from the fear of breast cancer. We now need to raise more than £5 million a year to fund our pioneering research programme.

How you can help – take up the Breakthrough £1,000 Challenge

The idea behind Breakthrough's £1,000 Challenge is simple – we challenge our supporters to raise £1,000 for the charity. This can be done by any (legal!) means and over any period of time. The names of £1,000 Challengers who achieve this target are displayed permanently at the Breakthrough Research Centre. Over 2,000 men and women have taken up – and met – the £1,000 Challenge. Some of them are featured in this book. Between them they have raised over £4 million for Breakthrough's vital research. Why don't you join them?

To register as a £1,000 Challenger or make a donation to Breakthrough, please call 020 7405 5111, visit www.breakthrough.org.uk or write to Breakthrough Breast Cancer, PO Box 8138, Halesowen B63 3FH.

Thank you for your support.